PRAISE FOR GAINING

"Liu exposes many myths surrounding eating disorders . . . She fleshes out facts and statistics with her personal interviews, making this book poignant even for those who have not suffered from an eating disorder."

—*Publishers Weekly*

"The beauty of Aimee Liu's brilliantly researched book is right there in the title. There *is* life after eating disorders, and Liu writes about that life with unflinching candor, exceptional insight, and remarkable bravery . . . Liu gives us a unique and provocative look at recovery . . . This is a groundbreaking work that's a must-read for anyone who has struggled with food or weight but didn't quite understand why."

—Lori Gottlieb, author of
Stick Figure: A Diary of My Former Self

"This book is the most sensitive, insightful, and beautifully crafted connection I have seen of personal experience with what scientists know about eating disorders. It is rich in emotion, understanding of human interaction, and lessons on culture, weight, and eating."

—Kelly D. Brownell, PhD
professor of psychology, epidemiology,
and public health, and director, Rudd Center
for Food Policy and Obesity, Yale University

*more . . .*

"GAINING is an engaging and incredibly insightful book . . . will hopefully encourage readers to examine their own lives and consider making changes that will contribute to their long-term health . . . and will encourage researchers and clinicians to continue to question what is meant by 'recovery' and how it can best be achieved."

—Renee Rienecke Hoste, PhD,
Academy for Eating Disorders Forum

"Valuable . . . a careful deconstruction of eating disorders . . . a solid resource."

—*Booklist*

<gaining>

---

the truth about life after
eating disorders

Aimee Liu

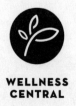

**WELLNESS
CENTRAL**

NEW YORK   BOSTON

"Green" by Leslie McGrath was originally published in *Nimrod*, Spring/Summer 2006, vol. 49, no. 2.

Wellness Central
Hachette Book Group USA
237 Park Avenue
New York, NY 10017

Visit our Web site at www.HachetteBookGroupUSA.com.

Printed in the United States of America

Originally published in hardcover by Hachette Book Group USA.

First Trade Edition: January 2008
10 9 8 7 6 5 4 3 2 1

Wellness Central is an imprint of Grand Central Publishing.
The Wellness Central name and logo is a trademark of Hachette Book Group USA, Inc.

ISBN 978-0-446-69482-7 (pbk.)
LCCN: 2006928995

Book design by Giorgetta Bell McRee

For Carolyn and Deborah,

in hope, awe, and friendship

Contents

III. A WIDER WORLD: *Consumer Society and Body Image*

Author's Note

THIS BOOK IS A PLEA. Back in the 1960s and 1970s, when I was suffering from anorexia nervosa, it was assumed that recovery could be measured in pounds. To the extent it existed at all, treatment for eating disorders was in its infancy. I did not receive treatment, and as I now recognize, my psychological recovery took decades. Today, fortunately, the landscape has changed. Skilled and gifted therapists who specialize in these disorders practice throughout the world. New scientific advances in treatment are occurring every day. Most important, these disorders are no longer treated as problems of eating and weight alone; they are recognized as signals of deeper distress. And while healthful nutrition is a vital step, it is no longer mistaken for the ultimate cure. My plea—to parents, doctors, teachers, coaches, and especially to those with a history of eating disorders—is to take the warning signal seriously. Get the professional help you need to decode it and resolve, or at least learn to manage, the true causes of distress, not merely the symptoms.

Some excellent eating disorders programs are mentioned in this book. Others can be located through the resources listed in the appendices. If someone you care about is signaling an alarm by starving herself or bingeing and purging, this book can help you understand what is happening beneath the surface. I hope it will also help you gain new insight into the process of recovery. But no book is a replacement for treatment. Please heed the warning, and seek help now.

Because I believe anorexia and bulimia to be syndromes that encompass far more than disordered eating, I am uneasy with the common usage of the terms *anorexic* and *bulimic* as body-centered nouns. Human beings are far too complicated to be summed up by any single word, particularly one that focuses on physical appearance or illness. Recovery is all about moving beyond such limitations. Nevertheless, in order to overcome any problem, we must first admit we *have* that problem. We must face it, examine it honestly, and learn how to manage it. That process of overcoming is the subject of this book. In this context, then, I use the terms *anorexic* and *bulimic* as shorthand, but advisedly, the way an author of a book about diabetes might refer to diabetics. I do not mean to imply that these disorders wholly define anyone. However, the alternative would be long, unwieldy sentences punctuated by "individuals who suffer from . . . ," which would distract and obscure instead of clarifying the substance of the book. The same reasoning governs my use of terms like *perfectionist, borderline,* or *avoidant.* These are all important aspects of identity; they are not the sum of identity.

Finally, a note about the people you will meet in these pages. Except for those who have written about their experiences themselves, or who gave me explicit permission, all names and identifying details of my interviews have been changed to protect their privacy. Many of their stories were painful to recount. All, ultimately, were inspiring. This book is a testament to these individuals' courage, honesty, and generosity.

Introduction

To Gain Is Good

gain (gān) *vi.* **1.** to make progress, improve or advance, as in health or career **2.** to acquire wealth or profit **3.** to increase in weight, gravity, or substance **4.** to increase in speed **5.** to win competitive advantage **6.** to move forward in time **7.** to mature or age

To GAIN IS GOOD. We gain confidence as we grow, status and health as we prosper, and—so we hope—wisdom as we age. A gain of intimacy is essential for love, of toughness for survival. By definition, gaining is a source of pleasure and progress. Why, then, do so many women (and, increasingly, men) confound the meaning of this simple, satisfying word with shame and dread? Weight is the obvious culprit but misleading, since those who fear gaining the most often have the least weight to lose. It's not really fat they fear, either, despite what they may say. It's all those positive, powerful gains that fulfill their deeper hungers. Some tell themselves they don't deserve a lover who can make them laugh. Others fear any promotion that involves responsibility. Still others instinctively distrust anyone who befriends them. The greatest fear, however, is that gaining will expose some shameful inner truth. It's not about the numbers on the scale. Deep down, we all know that.

Three decades ago, when I was in my young twenties, I wrote a memoir, *Solitaire*, in which I attempted to explain the horror of gaining that consumed my own adolescence. At thirteen I'd declared war on appetite and adopted discipline, abstinence, and self-punishment as my guiding principles. True, this war did seem to begin with a terror of food and weight. I would stretch a cookie for a month by eating it in crumbs, dissect brussels sprouts one leaf at a time, sip a spoonful of yogurt as if it were scalding soup. I spent up to four hours a day walking, cycling, and doing calisthenics. Eventually, I also denied myself friendship on the grounds that it might put temptation in my way. My weight dropped from 130 at age thirteen, when I reached my adult height of five foot seven, to 98 the following year. I could clamp my knees together and slide a fist between my thighs with room to spare. Still, I berated myself in front of the mirror as I stepped on and off and on the scale: "You are one fat slob." For seven years I cultivated my phobia of gaining; then in 1979 I pretended not only that I understood why but also that I was cured.

Nowhere in the pages of *Solitaire* did I name my obsession. That's because, as far as I knew growing up in the sixties and early seventies, it had no name. I lived in the affluent, mostly white town of Greenwich, Connecticut, where hunger was a problem seen only on nightly news reports from the Third World. And though the boyishly gaunt supermodel Twiggy began appearing in *Vogue* in 1966, when I started dieting the following year her bone thinness was still too controversial to be considered iconic. The prevailing standards of beauty, however, were only marginally more substantial. Audrey Hepburn—Hollywood's ideal for thin chic since the fifties—may have been described as gamine rather than boyish, but her 34-20-34 measurements still were more childlike than womanly. My mother, who styled herself in Hepburn's image, bemoaned every pound she herself gained, and when I started putting on weight with puberty and requested a bathroom scale and diet books for Christmas, she willingly obliged.

At school, as the pounds slipped off my body, I detected envy from other girls. This was new and intoxicating. I'd always been the teacher's pet, a conscientious daughter, a straight-A student; the last to be picked for any team in PE, and the girl no boy would think of asking out. Now even the popular girls complimented me on my willpower. Soon I had competition. Our sophomore homecoming princess dropped nearly forty pounds in two months. My best friend joined me for lunches that consisted solely of black coffee. Another of my classmates shrank so drastically that her skin grew a fine layer of furry hair, called *lanugo*, which was her body's attempt to protect her against hypothermia due to the loss of body fat. Eventually this girl was hospitalized for forced feeding, and months later returned to school so bloated I hardly recognized her. Her example might have warned the rest of us to put on some weight. Instead, we went into hiding under extra sweatshirts, baggy pants, and layered jackets, disguising our thinness to safeguard it.

Although few of us were diagnosed back then, my wasted classmates and I all met the clinical criteria for anorexia nervosa: we'd purposely reduced our weight to less than 85 percent of a normal minimum for our age and height; we suffered a phobic fear of becoming fat; we had a distorted view of our body shape and size, insisting—always—that we were not thin enough; weight loss caused us to cease, or never begin, menstruating. Some of us had restricting anorexia, meaning that we achieved thinness exclusively by fasting or cutting calories. Others had exercise anorexia and manically worked off the pounds without strenuous dieting, or binge-purge anorexia, meaning they sometimes grossly overate but then made themselves vomit.

There were also girls in my school who were not underweight but, we all knew, were purging. Some of them boasted

about it. We were in the back of a station wagon on the way to
an eighth-grade basketball game when Tricia, a round-faced girl
I'd known since kindergarten who giggled as she talked, announced that she'd found the "solution" to gaining. Though she
probably weighed about 110, I was already anorexic and
thought of her as chunky, so I doubted her solution worked. I
also judged it disgusting and weak, since my weight loss, to that
point, had been accomplished solely through self-discipline.
But I began to notice after that how certain other girls, too,
would load up on grilled cheese sandwiches or pizza at lunch,
then scurry to the lavatory before their next class; how they developed chipmunk cheeks, blotchy skin, and dull hair. They
sounded hoarse and had teeth as stained as long-time smokers.
Some slipped each other squares of Ex-Lax—not realizing that
laxatives purge less than 10 percent of calories consumed and
apparently not caring that laxative abuse can cause excruciat-
ing gastrointestinal damage, cardiac arrest, and death. The girls
who binged and purged tended, for reasons I could not then
fathom, to be more outgoing than those of us who fasted. They
led cheers at the football games while we hid in the library, but
they were no less shackled by the fear of gaining.

Our parents, meanwhile, met our strange behavior with a variety of responses. Some of these executives and homemakers,
nurses, ministers, and stockbrokers worried that we were sick.
Some denied there was any problem. Many blamed us. Medical
doctors, after all, found no illness to explain our weight loss,
and in a community as prosperous and image conscious as ours,
few parents would entertain the possibility that something
might be psychologically wrong with their children—or, by extension, with themselves. My fellow dieters and I had always
been compliant, helpful, studious, and orderly; and except for
our stubborn refusal to eat, we retained those qualities. Even at
our thinnest, we excelled in our studies. Many of us were talented artists, writers, musicians, or dancers. Our teachers
praised us and our parents boasted about us even as they

lamented or rebuked us for our obstinacy. We represented a paradox: Why would young women who stood to gain so much in life try so hard to destroy themselves?

In fact, our dread of gaining in life was far greater than our fear of fat. Most of us denied our sexual maturity, and we shrank from power and authority. "Oh no," we'd say, "I could never—" You name it: run for class president, conduct the orchestra, stand up to our parents, lead a protest, say no to a boy who wanted sex or enjoy sex even if—perish the thought!—we actually wanted it, too. Instead, we pulled deep into ourselves, away from conflict and external risk, in search of a zone of psychological safety that would make us feel untouchable. On the rare occasions when someone asked why we did this, we'd mumble something about not feeling good enough. We didn't feel we'd earned the right to be respected or listened to. Self-denial: that's what made us feel right with the world.

By my twisted logic, gaining and losing became so thoroughly confused that I sabotaged even gains that filled me with pride. At fifteen, I was accepted by Wilhelmina, one of the world's foremost modeling agencies. Photographers pegged my look as "fresh and young." I made the cover of *American Girl* and had spreads in *Seventeen, Coed,* and *Ingenue* magazines. I hoped modeling would pay for college, and at first it seemed it might. But my new occupation fueled my obsession with my weight to the point where anorexia actually undermined my career. I lost so much weight that at seventeen, I no longer fit the clothes I was supposed to showcase; the career I'd been so thrilled by was over before I could reap its rewards.

Then, in 1970, I was admitted into Yale University's third-ever class of freshmen women. Though eager to leave home, where my weight had become a source of constant friction, I clung to my high school boyfriend, an art major one year ahead of me. He, conveniently for me, believed that fasting, sleep deprivation, and grueling exercise had spiritual benefits. I loved him for keeping me company in my compulsions, even if his rationale sometimes eluded me. My second day on campus I moved into his dorm room and for the next year rarely left his side. We took the same classes, ate lettuce together, shared the same small circle of friends. He shielded me from other men, and we nurtured each other's emotional dependence. It took me more than two years to realize the relationship could not last.

Then I had belatedly to face the problem of defining myself. I could continue like the dozen other lost waifs who drifted hungrily across campus with heads down and eyes averted, or I could look up and make a place for myself among the rest of my classmates—the ones who struck me as "normal." The variety of normalcy at Yale was daunting. This was a school where Russian choristers debated paradigm shifts and Keynesian economics during late night sessions at Naples Pizza; painters plotted ménages à trois with poets over beer at Rudy's; and young women from Trinidad and Watts argued the relative merits of careers with Citibank and the Rand Corporation over deviled eggs and sherry at masters' teas. To my mind, the classmates who juggled ideas, appetites, and prospects were nothing like me. They intimidated me. They overpowered me. But they also took me in, inviting my opinion, prodding me to relax. They taught me to act as if I knew who I was and what I wanted. When I graduated from college I weighed 110.

While it would be a serious overstatement to say that I felt comfortable in my enlarged body, I did believe the obsession that had dominated my adolescence was over. By the time I was twenty-three, I had gained another ten pounds. I had an apartment in New York City and worked as a flight attendant while trying to launch a writing career. One day I came across an article in *Vogue* about girls who purposely starved themselves to concentration camp thinness, and I learned for the first time that the syndrome which had dominated my teens actually had a medical name.

I devoured the few books that had then been published about anorexia nervosa—notably Hilde Bruch's groundbreaking *The Golden Cage* and *Eating Disorders: Obesity, Anorexia Nervosa, and the Person Within*. Bruch described eating disorders as reactions to experience—to sexual abuse, for instance, or a narcissistic mother or pressure from a gymnastics coach to lose weight. Anorexics were victims of circumstance, she implied, the way consumptives were victims of bacteria. They were also victims of the illusion that losing weight would make them special. How well I knew that illusion! One of my primary goals in fasting had been to set myself apart. In my journals I'd often used that very word: *special*. In retrospect, however, I suspected what I'd actually been seeking was something far less grandiose. I wasn't trying to prove my superiority so much as my *authenticity*. As far back as I could remember, I'd felt ill equipped for convention and longed to follow a path of my own making. In my teens I imagined anorexia to be such a path. In fact, though, what had seemed to me an original pursuit had turned me into a *stereotypical* anorexic.

If I had realized this error while still a teenager, would I have sought a more positive way to frame my individuality? I suspected I would at least have become more self-aware, and that might have spared me some of those wasted years. By the same reasoning, I thought my story might serve as a cautionary tale for younger girls.

Unlike most of the narratives and self-help books about anorexia nervosa that would follow, *Solitaire* did not include harrowing scenes of hospitalization or therapy sessions, for the simple reason that I, like most of my anorexic classmates, was never treated. My goal, then, was not to sensationalize but to chronicle the typical anorexic experience, which at the time I believed to be a product of late-twentieth-century adolescence and a culture obsessed with thin women. I portrayed myself as someone who had been drawn into a dangerous trend but managed to correct my course before it was too late. There was just one problem: as I hinted in *Solitaire*'s postscript, "the piec～ ～ the puzzle" were still in play. I'd resumed eating, yes. I' gained those lost pounds. But what I could not bring myself to admit in the memoir was that my "recovery" had set off a whole new wave of self-abuse.

As I began to gain weight I'd become secretly and seriously bulimic. I also drank too much, slept with men I never intended to see a second time, and pretended not to care. It didn't occur to me that these "bad behaviors," so common as to seem typical of my peers, might in my case constitute another face of anorexia. I did realize that for seven years I'd pantomimed my anxiety and alienation by shrinking my body. I knew this show of discomfort had done nothing to identify, much less resolve, the actual sources of discomfort. Yet I now wanted to believe that gaining weight was enough to make me feel normal. Neither in *Solitaire* nor in my own mind could I explain how that process would happen. What did "normal" even feel like? How did "normal" think? Anorexia had so distorted my perspective that I had no idea. In retrospect, I realize that I simply replaced anorexia with more conventional and less conspicuous, but perhaps no less damaging, methods of acting out what I refused to admit I was feeling. At the time, I saw no connection. I pretended, even to myself, that I felt fine.

From readers I received notes of thanks. *Solitaire* had broken the silence that, in those days, still shrouded the subject of eating disorders. Most of these young women reported that they were now recovering, starting careers and, in some cases, families of their own. But their letters spoke of the same unfinished business I was denying. One reader wrote, "Did you ever find yourself relapsing into bingeing, in spite of your changed mindset? Or did you find that once you had broken the cycle, there was no going back? Did you feel tempted at times to retreat to that behavior, or was it not even a thought or issue anymore?" Another asked, "Do you still obsess about making mistakes? Do you ever worry that your kids might become anorexic?" Gaining weight had not resolved my readers' history of anorexia any more than it had mine.

This was true, too, for my classmates who'd had eating disorders. As the years passed I'd spot them at reunions, just as I used to across the quad, and note who was still—or again—painfully thin or shrinking behind her husband, running herself down in conversation, or micromanaging the table settings while others debated global politics. When we compared notes, I learned that many of these women—and a few men—were taking antidepressants. Most still struggled for distance from their parents. And virtually all habitually minimized their accomplishments and ambitions, a pattern that tended to bewilder and annoy their friends, colleagues, and families. These were dogged, driven workers, but no matter how many degrees or titles they'd earned, they still apologized for not doing enough, not trying or working harder. Even at thirty or forty, few could articulate what they "really" wanted in life. It was as if the face in the mirror belonged to a stranger, while the person who ought to appear remained in hiding.

For two decades I employed a typically anorexic strategy to deal with these observations: I declared myself an expert without acknowledging I still had a problem. *Solitaire* was the beginning of this pseudotherapy. I went on to write self-help books on love, success, parenthood, and codependence. My coauthors were renowned doctors and psychologists who became my friends, yet I never once consulted them about my own history or insecurities. Treating myself as cured and fully in control, I married and raised two boys, became an activist for equal rights and literary freedom, turned to fiction and wrote three novels. Then, after twenty years, my marriage began to unravel.

When my husband asked me what I wanted from him, I said I didn't know. I said he was too controlling, he wanted me to read his mind. I had no idea what he was thinking. I hated that he ate ice cream straight out of the carton, or the way he left his dirty gym clothes around the bathroom, and his habit of eating a half pound of nuts while watching the play-offs and calling that dinner. Finally he retaliated: my petty insults were bullshit. A fight, he could handle, but not this incessant needling. He couldn't stand the way I left notes instead of talking to him directly. Did I realize half the time I spent at my desk all I was doing was hiding? Why couldn't I just say whatever the hell it was I wanted? I cried. He yelled. I cheated. Then he did. I groped for distraction. I wanted some *thing*, some external change that I could pretend would solve our problems. I began compulsively house hunting.

Month after month I read the real estate section as if it held a magic formula. I joined the Tuesday caravans and patrolled the streets of west Los Angeles every Sunday for open houses. I toured mansions, bungalows, haciendas, tract homes, villas, and beach shacks. I was voracious in my searching, indiscriminate and unstoppable. Leaving the house in which my marriage was sputtering and moving us to a new "dream house" soon took on the same obsessive allure for me at forty-six that losing weight and moving into a tighter, leaner body had held for me at fourteen.

Finally I settled on a home. A towering sweet gum shaded the front circle drive, and four palm trees swayed above the wide back lawn and guesthouse; the master bedroom had a fireplace and cathedral ceilings; French doors opened from the family room onto a breezy lanai and swimming pool; our teenage son (my stepson by this time was grown) would have a whole suite to himself downstairs. Built in 1920, the house offered space, quiet, charm, and a sense of history—everything I thought we needed. My husband disagreed. At least the home he'd bought with his former wife—an expanded Spanish bungalow in which he and I had lived for two decades next to a commercial alley with nightly patrols of police helicopters thrumming overhead—didn't require any more work. "My" home needed rewiring, a new roof, removal of several walls, and a number of fundamental plumbing improvements. "You make it sound like a teardown," I protested. I believed whatever the cost, the potential merited the effort of remodeling. I thought the same thing about our marriage.

I rationalized: my husband's high-pressure job was to blame for our separate bedtimes, but it also would finance our dream house; my passion for real estate bordered on hysteria, but it would pay off when we made our move; our thirteen-year-old son didn't want to move any more than his father did, but he'd soon be seduced by the pool at the new place, the friends down the block. After weeks of backing and forthing, my husband countered with his solution. We'd buy the house. I could do what I wanted with it, move where I wanted to. He was staying put.

We bought the house and started both individual and couples therapy with Dr. Gold, who resembled W. C. Fields; talked like Groucho Marx; and offered the wisdom of Freud, Jung, Erikson, the Upanishads, and the Talmud. For the next four months, while I reconstructed walls and wiring, Gold prompted me and my husband to deconstruct our long history together, take stock of ourselves at midlife, bring up old grievances and expose new ones. I thought we were making as much progress in therapy as I was with the electrician. But on the day my son and I moved, I finally had to face the truth: I had left my husband, and he didn't know if he wanted me enough to follow.

My response was as unexpected as it was reflexive. I pretended—still—that I had everything under control. And I stopped eating.

As I'd hoped, my son soon adjusted to the move, but now he spent every waking minute, when he wasn't at school or on the soccer field, with his friends down the block. I didn't protest. I could understand, under the circumstances, why he'd want to steer clear of both his parents. But with no one around for dinner, there was no one to notice that I skipped it—or that I weighed myself incessantly, or that I would go out for a walk and not return for hours. Only I knew what I was doing. The rationale was as familiar as a school yard dare. If I could endure—even embrace—the hunger for food, then I could surely survive the suddenly searing hunger for my husband and child. Just as I used to at age fourteen, I took solace in the numbers on the bathroom scale.

Now, I was a long way from too thin, and my retreat to hunger took me nowhere near the 90-pound danger zone of my adolescence. The risk in this new slippage was not physical but psychological. No matter who denied my existence, I could deny myself first. If I took out my anger on nobody else, I could still take it out on myself. No matter how much or what I lost, I could always reassure myself by wanting nothing. "It's the divorce diet," I cracked when Dr. Gold noticed I was losing weight. He often made fun of his own ample borscht belly. I thought he'd appreciate the joke.

But Gold was not amused. Instead, he urged me to examine the role hunger and my response to it had played in my marriage—and, more important, in my life. This hunger soon became the focus of our sessions. We talked about my reluctance to wake up in the morning; the years I had spent rewriting a novel that never seemed to satisfy me; my continuing compulsion to paint the bathrooms, reorganize the kitchen cabinets, perfect the appearance of this new house even at the expense of my marriage. There was nothing new in any of this. I remembered scouring the kitchen sink for hours during a visit to my grandmother's farm when she was dying and I was dieting down to 95 pounds. Twenty years of marriage, parenthood, stepparenthood, and multiple careers had done little to change my basic instincts. Dr. Gold understood and made me understand. Basic instincts might shape our behavior and even determine the course of our lives, but only if we *choose*—actively or by default—to give them this power.

Divorce was not a foregone conclusion. My husband had embarked on a parallel course of self-examination, and Dr. Gold warned each of us against second-guessing the other. The focus, at least initially, had to be our selves. And I had to admit that whatever had made me go hungry in my teens was still gnawing at me in my forties. It had nothing to do with my husband. This realization, along with Gold's imperative, prompted me to stop retreating into self-denial and start, belatedly, to study it.

I read the many books that had been published about eating disorders since *Solitaire*. I contacted my classmates who had been anorexic or bulimic in high school and college. I looked up women who'd written to me after *Solitaire* was published, raised the subject at women's luncheons and book groups, posted a call for interviewees on my Web site, consulted eating disorder specialists and researchers. I was determined to find out what created the acute anxiety that seemed to underscore these disorders—an anxiety of identity, of ambivalence and desire. Why did so many former anorexics and bulimics suffer from lifelong depression? Were people who had received therapy more confident and self-accepting than those who recovered on their own? How did having children affect them? Divorce? Prozac? Why did so many of us in middle age still act as if the word *gaining* were a curse? Was it simply because we were women? Because we were brainwashed by Calvin Klein lingerie ads? Were our struggles with appetite the same as those of people who compulsively overate or chronically dieted without going to extremes? Or was something else going on?

Soon I had dozens of interviews and even more secondhand stories. It turned out I wasn't the only one who used to watch my starving and bulimic classmates as if they were sibling rivals. Lori Gottlieb, whose memoir *Stick Figure* chronicled her passage through anorexia at eleven, recalled girls at school who ran compulsively at midnight, in blizzards, or through downpours; who ate nothing but broth and lentils; or who made three trips to the bathroom during every meal. "Not only could I name every one of them today," Lori told me, "but I've met some women as adults, knowing nothing about them except the way they talk and act, and I'll think, they had an eating disorder, and sure enough, they did—twenty years ago." One of my older interviewees remembered a girl who used to throw up in her dorm bathroom at Vassar in the 1950s. Several women told me about grandfathers who were lifelong anorexics. Many had deduced that their mothers, sisters, aunts, and/or grandmothers had eating disorders, though they were never diagnosed. And an alarming number of former anorexics and bulimics had children who showed the same tendencies.

These stories, along with the latest research findings, demolished Hilde Bruch's stereotype of the eating disordered as modern rich white girls whose parents and coaches trained them to be sick. They also persuaded me that culture alone does not cause obsession with food and weight. People with histories of anorexia and bulimia tend to be temperamentally different from each other as well as from people who never develop an eating disorder or who compulsively overeat. Concentrating on anorexia and bulimia because these were the eating disorders I knew, I tried to look deeper into these distinctions. I spoke with men as well as women who ranged in age from twenty to sixty. Several of my interviewees had experienced either their first symptoms or relapse in their forties. Some were gay, some straight; some married, some single; some wealthy, some struggling financially. They included Jews, Christians, Buddhists, atheists, and agnostics. I met a Puerto Rican artist who had been bulimic into her thirties; a Cuban writer who began bingeing and purging on chocolate after he quit drinking; an anorexic, half African American, half Chinese, who for ten years never ate more than a slice of tomato and a lettuce leaf for lunch; a five-foot-nine law student from Bombay who became obsessed with running and dieting as he entered his last year of graduate school and in two months sliced his weight from 160 to 110.

The people I interviewed were also professionally diverse: authors, artists, actors, filmmakers, architects, librarians, hospital administrators, doctors, and insurance adjusters. Among my former classmates, Yvonne Anderson teaches comparative religion, Candace Lunt is a magazine editor, Joyce Maynard is a journalist and novelist, and Kim Olensky came back from her second major anorexic relapse to earn a master's in counseling that she might help others avoid the psychological traps she had repeatedly set for herself. Kim's career path turned out to be a popular one. Several of the therapists I consulted as experts had also once struggled with eating disorders themselves.

I was astonished, then, when even those who were veterans of therapy said that much of what we discussed they'd never shared with anyone before. They hadn't made the connection between their early compulsion to suppress hunger and their later extramarital affairs. They hadn't thought about how their punishing workouts at fourteen had translated into workaholism and career burnout at forty. They hadn't noticed how instinctively they downplayed the pleasure of food and taste when feeding their children—just as they still denied themselves that pleasure—or how they now held back their emotions the same way they used to hold back their physical appetites. It became evident that traces of our eating disorders have been present throughout our lives. Concerns about weight, diet, and physical appearance notwithstanding, we have always struggled to feel at home in our bodies, our relationships, and our emotions. Even now, for most of us, power remains a source of ambivalence, intimacy an arena of doubt, and passion a tantalizing threat. Gaining perspective is an ongoing challenge. It is also an enormously liberating process.

In the work of renowned British child development expert D. W. Winnicott I found a way to visualize the problem of personal perspective. Winnicott observed that everyone experiences three interlocking lives, which together shape his or her individual sense of identity. The first is an inner life of emotions, sensation, and imagination. The second is lived through relationships with family, lovers, and friends. The third is one's experience of culture and society through, for example, the media, politics, and work. Ideally, these three lives develop like concentric circles, with one's inner self securely centered, strengthened and supported by close relations, and so able to respond independently to culture. This kind of self-centeredness results in a person comfortable in her skin, who knows how she feels when her stomach growls, what she wants from her husband, and why she changes the channel when she sees a beer commercial in which ultrathin, perfectly sculpted young women are playing volleyball in bikinis for the amusement of a bunch of leering, fully dressed men. But people who develop eating disorders often live "out of order." They have difficulty trusting their instincts. Their relationships make them feel anxious instead of supported. So instead of engaging with the outer world from a position of internal strength, they substitute the demands of media culture for their core beliefs—living, in effect, outside in. This is how teenage girls come to believe they must look like those bikini-clad volleyball players in order to feel normal; how Phi Beta Kappas can feel compelled to shrink their healthy size-10 bodies down to size 0; how middle-aged women dying of cancer can say—and mean it—"Well, at least I'm thin."

Gaining back a full, healthy life in the wake of an eating disorder is largely a process of restoring these three realms of experience to their rightful order. The first, most important, and in many cases ongoing challenge is to look beyond the surface of the person in the mirror. As University of New Mexico psychiatrist Joel Yager told me, "Know thyself in a very profound Greek way. What is your biology? What is your calling? How are you built? Study your temperament. Be respectful of it." The second stage involves reexamining and adjusting relationships with families, lovers, and friends. "You're not going to turn yourself into someone you aren't," Yager explained, "and nobody should try to turn you into someone you're not built to be." With enough self-awareness, we can rebuild or form new relationships around trust instead of judgment. Then, aided by this genuine support, we can renegotiate our responses to our culture and society from a position of personal confidence instead of emptiness. When what we do, want, and admire is shaped by a strong sense of self that operates from the inside out, we gain true power over our lives. These three stages of gaining, then, correspond to the sections in which this book is organized.

As I met with the men and women whose stories fill these pages and we compared our oddly parallel experiences and idiosyncrasies, a funny thing happened: our lives seemed to fall into the perspective we had long been seeking. Anxieties that we'd thought shameful—terror of argument, wallflower shyness, or fear of orgasm, to name just a few—turned out to be problems most of us shared and that had singularly unshameful, often biochemical causes. Experiences that once seemed insurmountable—parental violence, childhood molestation, deep and chronic depression—helped to explain not only who we were as individuals but also why as a group we behaved in so many of the same ways. And as we connected all these dots, some of our most persistent tendencies—to manically clean each pot in the kitchen or color code our closets, to time our workout sessions to the second or lie awake berating ourselves for errors in conversation that no one else even noticed—finally began to seem absurd. When I asked Chicago homemaker Lucy Romanello, who had been anorexic nearly thirty years earlier, how her husband felt about her ongoing compulsion to vacuum, she earnestly defended herself: "Well, I try not to clean right out from under him!" When I laughed, it took her by surprise, but a moment later she saw the humor as well as the lesson glimmering in her remark. The time had come to stop this charade of self-control. We all had so much to gain.

Part One

KNOW THYSELF

Temperamental Truths

1

CONNECTING THE DOTS

A Genetic Link

> When I write of hunger, I am really writing
> about love and the hunger for it, and warmth
> and the love of it and the hunger for it . . . and
> then the warmth and richness and fine reality of
> hunger satisfied . . . and it is all one.
> —M. F. K. Fisher

MY FRIEND CAROL, CALLING FROM SANTA FE, sounded elated as she told me her news: after thirty years, she'd finally located our high school classmate Candy Lunt. The last time either of us had seen Candy was at graduation, when she weighed less than 80 pounds. Shortly thereafter, her family left Greenwich. The possible implications of her continuing absence from our alumni directory had haunted both Carol and me.

"You should be a bounty hunter!" I said. "Where is she?"

"I spotted her name on the masthead of *Forbes*."

"No!"

"I called her. Aimee, she still talks in that half whisper from the back of her throat, low and deep—you remember?"

Barely. What I remembered more, at least at the end, was her silence.

"She's an editor," Carol raced on. "She lives in Manhattan with her daughter. Somehow, she's *okay*."

I wondered. As I'd recently discovered, there was a big difference between survival and well-being. "Was she glad to hear from you?"

"She and Ruby are coming to the ranch for a visit next week. Can you come, too?"

"You couldn't stop me," I said.

Such invitations were characteristic of Carol. She had been diagnosed with non-Hodgkin's lymphoma fourteen years earlier, at thirty-four, and during her first remission she'd launched a personal campaign to track down as many as possible of her "disappeareds"—friends she'd lost through the passage of time. I'd been back in Carol's orbit for twelve years now, and between her life with cancer and my marital separation four months earlier, we were closer than we'd ever been in school. But I was surprised by Candy's quick response after all these years.

"By the way," Carol said before hanging up, "she calls herself Candace now."

So, I thought as I packed for the trip from Los Angeles, Candy's taken a grown-up name. I found this disorienting. I didn't know Candace Lunt, whereas I'd first met Candy in third grade, when we were nine years old. We joined the Beach Boys fan club together. At my house in those preanorexic days, we baked coffee cake. At hers we ate hot dogs. I remember even as a child finding her ranch-style tract house forbidding. My childhood home was like a museum, filled with Chinese heirlooms—my father's ancestry—and temple rubbings, carved icons, and brass work acquired during my family's two years in India. While these treasures reflected my parents' pride of possession, dust did tend to accumulate. The Lunts, too, had lived abroad—in Mexico—but in their house you could see the vacuum tracks in the white carpets, hear the click of the wall clock bounce off the spotless kitchen Formica. Candy's mother and mine both worked, which in suburban Connecticut in the sixties was unusual. Mine imported hand-loomed textiles from India. Hers, a trim, prematurely white-haired woman whom I never once saw smile, was a dental hygienist. My father commuted into Manhattan to run the guided tour service at the United Nations, while Mr. Lunt was a senior vice president with Ford Motors. Candy had two older brothers to my one. And she was smaller, freckled, quiet. Even before she had braces, she always covered her mouth when she laughed.

By senior year Candy was one of the most withdrawn girls in our school. That was 1970. More than three hundred thousand American kids were fighting in Vietnam, and that spring the National Guard opened fire on antiwar students at Kent State. While Kate Millett had just published *Sexual Politics*, most of the girls in our class still wore miniskirts and painted their lips with Yardley Slickers. Candy, however, shunned makeup. She used her long ginger-colored hair as a screen. She avoided both our school's peace protests and the senior prom.

I arrived a day ahead of Candace at the restored adobe farmhouse Carol shared with her husband, Wayne. Carol and I had known each other since sophomore year in high school when I was just starting my modeling career. Carol back then lived in peasant blouses, blue jeans, and clogs. She always seemed to be baking a carrot cake or making joyous, boldly hued silk screens styled after the artist Sister Corita. She also knew how to fly a Cessna and shoot her dad's Smith & Wesson. Naturally slender and small-boned, Carol had never so much as flirted with anorexia nervosa, but she held a unique attraction for those of us who did. This was partly because she never seemed to judge us, but mostly because we wished we could be like her. Now, at forty-seven she was an accomplished graphic designer, painter, and horsewoman. She lived in cowboy boots and kept paints and pastels in her kitchen next to the sugar and olive oil. She was still my favorite role model.

We brought each other up-to-date on the respective states of my marriage and Carol's illness, both in flux with uncertain outcomes. Then Carol said, "Candace's divorce was just finalized." The two of us, she intimated, should find plenty to talk about. And since Carol was weakened from her latest round of chemo, I would be making the hour drive to pick up Candace and her daughter at the Albuquerque airport.

As I hovered by the security checkpoint I wondered what I was looking for. I'd gained more than thirty pounds since high school, and current friends seeing my old modeling pictures would bluntly ask, "That's *you?*" Surely Candy would be equally transformed. But my thoughts kept sliding back to my last images of her. Seventeen years old, she sat alone in the corner of the cafeteria making a half hour meal out of a six-ounce container of plain yogurt. Though in many ways her mirror image, I rarely spoke to her. By then, we pitied each other. We also admired each other. We knew each other's secrets without knowing the details, and so, on a subliminal level, we feared each other.

"Aimee?" The voice came softly from my right. I turned and immediately recognized my friend from third grade. She still wore her hair long and straight, no makeup to hide her freckles; and her eyes were that same cerulean blue: quiet, steady, yet voracious.

When we hugged, her grip felt healthy, her body trim but solid. She smelled like Breck shampoo. So did her daughter, Ruby—a wary, dark-eyed child still sleepy from her nap on the plane. Ruby was the same age Candy and I had been when we first met.

On the drive to Santa Fe, Candace told me she and Ruby had moved to lower Manhattan three years earlier from San Francisco and were only now settling in. She glanced toward the backseat. Ruby, she said, was one of those kids who have just three friends and know everything about them from how they arranged their socks to what they muttered in their sleep. It hadn't been any easier for Ruby to find such friends in New York than it had been for her to deal with her parents' divorce.

"How long were you married?"

"Fifteen years." Her ex-husband, Candace explained, was her opposite: he'd voted for Bush, attended church, had working-class parents who drank, and was happy to cruise for a year between jobs—largely because Candace covered the bills. Before disappearing, he'd cleaned out her bank account. Candace had nearly lost her own job while fighting her husband in court—to little avail. She'd also lost twenty pounds—the first relapse into anorexia since college.

"The divorce diet," I said, not joking.

She nodded. Five years later, she'd regained the weight but was still struggling to sort out what had gone wrong in the marriage. "I tried to tell him, 'I'm like a plant and you're overwatering me,'" she said. "But he was too needy, and when he couldn't have all my attention, he turned vengeful."

It seemed to me she was giving her ex more credit than he deserved, but I knew from my own experience there had to be more to the story. "It falls into the category of 'be careful what you wish for,'" I said when Candace asked about my separation. Superficially, my marriage had all the right ingredients. My husband was generous, smart, devoted to our sons, and more attractive to me with his silver hair at sixty than any man I'd dated in my twenties. Maybe the problem was the fourteen-year age gap. Maybe it was his latest business deal, which had turned him into a workaholic. Of course I'd never cared about the Lakers, and he couldn't stand to socialize, especially with my friends. Worse, we'd do anything to avoid honest confrontation . . . But all these were evasions. "I'm still sorting out my role in all this," I admitted. "But I guess the important realization is that I played one."

"You're ahead of the game," Candace said. "I didn't realize that until it was too late."

When we reached the ranch, the afternoon turned into a blur of activity as Carol showed off her painting and photography studios, and we played with the horses and dogs. We didn't settle down until evening, when Carol brought out a set of easy-bake mugs for us to paint at the large wooden table in the middle of her kitchen. As everyone got to work I felt like I'd landed back in art class in elementary school—the more so when I glanced up and saw Candace covering her mouth with her hand as she smiled at something Ruby had said. Carol drew hearts and horses, a miniature of the view from her window, with printed words of love. Ruby made free-form swirls, letting herself go. Candace created a meticulous, pointillist ocean of fishes. I stared at the surface of my cup.

I applied the marker. I erased the mark. A picture was supposed to present itself, but my mind was as blank as the clay. I stole another look at Candace's impeccable sea as Carol's husband, Wayne, strolled through the kitchen. He took one look at me and in his amused, laid-back way said, "Aimee. It's *only* a *mug*."

Candace threw me a look of sympathy. Carol frowned at Candace's mug. All those compulsively ordered dots. "This is supposed to be fun," Carol said.

Ruby grinned and held up her abstraction. "I'm having fun!"

We laughed, and I loosened up enough to deface my mug with a maze of inked leaves, but it wasn't fun for me.

When we talked about it later, Candace told me she often drew in points, trying to make pictures out of the negative space. "I guess it goes back to my failed attempts at therapy," she said. "They never connected the dots."

"What do you mean by *dots*?"

"You know. Weight and men, my body, my family." She described her longing to let loose. She felt she needed to make some enormous, meaningful gesture through her work or music. "But it's as if this impulse is gridlocked by the compulsion to always behave."

I felt this gridlock, too. In my bones. In that silly mug drawing. In my lifelong habit of biting my nails. I glanced across the table. Yes, Candace also chewed her nails, although, tellingly, she had succeeded in restricting herself to her left ring finger.

Was anorexia nervosa merely another symptom of this internal constraint? The more Candace and I talked, the more we did seem to have in common. Our similarities went way beyond where and when we were raised: we both dreaded making a mistake; both hated being the center of attention, even though we craved praise and needed to excel; we didn't laugh easily or openly or trust ourselves to relax. I imagined the two of us standing side by side, question marks tattooed on our foreheads.

That night I said to Candace, "If we went back and talked with the other women we knew who had eating disorders in high school and college, I think we'd find we all have more in common—even today—than we have with the rest of our classmates."

But Candace was not so sure. "Don't you think people change?"

"I think they can when they know what needs changing. Gaining weight was only a first step—for me, at least."

She studied her hands. Something I'd said seemed to pain her. But when she looked up, she said only, "I'd be interested in knowing . . . in hearing those stories."

I thought about asking to interview Candace right then, but Carol and Ruby pulled us in other directions. Besides, I was not yet sure what questions to ask. The skeptic in me warned that women who'd had eating disorders constituted a broad and diverse group. Their lives were affected by a multitude of factors, and if they appeared similar it was as likely because of shared culture as any innate parallel. But Candace's phrase "connect the dots" stayed with me long after I was back in LA. I kept remembering that look she'd shot me as we labored over our mugs, the two of us still holding back in a way no one else in the kitchen that night could understand.

In 1979, when I published *Solitaire*, anorexia nervosa was generally considered a recent phenomenon, and bulimia had just that year been named—by British psychiatrist Gerald Russell, from *bous*, meaning "ox" (read: "beastly") and *limos*, "hunger." In fact, neither disorder was new. In *Phthisiologia, or, A Treatise of Consumptions*, published in 1694, British physician Richard Morton wrote of a twenty-year-old girl who refused to eat, studied all the time, and looked "like a Skeleton only clad with Skin." Anorexia was named from the Greek *an*, meaning "lack of," and *orexis*, "appetite," by French physician Charles Lasègue in a paper documenting eight cases of willful fasting in 1873. And countless girls before 1979 practiced bulimia. Jane Fonda, for instance, learned this "secret" from a friend in boarding school in the 1950s: "We assumed we were the first people since the Romans to do this," she recalled in her memoir *My Life So Far*. Diana, Princess of Wales, admitted in 1997 that she'd begun bingeing and purging in the early 1970s; and her sister Sarah was hospitalized with binge-purge anorexia in 1975. Yet because the true scope of eating disorders wasn't recognized until the 1980s, most doctors treated such cases back then as mystifying oddities.

In 1978 in *The Golden Cage*, Hilde Bruch had painted the typical anorexic as a birdlike child "too plain and simple for the luxuries of her home, but also deprived of the freedom of doing what she truly wanted to do." Anorexia nervosa, Bruch suggested, was a symptom of arrested development caused by lack of parental encouragement. She identified overconscientious, overstudious, and compliant performance as a warning sign and noted that when patients first came to her, "they looked, acted, and sounded amazingly alike" even though they had widely differing backgrounds and included several boys. She rejected, however, any possibility that these kids might have looked, acted, or sounded alike *before* they got sick. The medical similarities, she argued, were due to the fact that these patients were all starving organisms. And the psychological and behavioral parallels were the result of coincidentally parallel family dynamics.

To explain why anorexia nervosa seemed so lopsidedly to affect middle- and upper-class girls, Bruch pointed to "the enormous emphasis that Fashion places on slimness" and the message delivered through advertising that women can be loved and respected only when slender. She also worried that the women's liberation movement of the 1960s, while expanding their opportunities, had intensified the pressure on teenage girls to prove themselves in arenas such as physics, soccer, debating . . . and bed, before they were ready. All this new freedom threatened to overwhelm the overconscientious, Bruch suggested, and some turned to hunger as an obsessional escape.

Feminist social critics deflected the blame by broadening it. In 1978 Susie Orbach declared that "Fat Is a Feminist Issue." In 1981 Kim Chernin described "the tyranny of slenderness" as "The Obsession" that our society imposes on women, primarily through the marketplace and media. The true villain in the feminist portrait of eating disorders was not the mother figure, and certainly not women's liberation, but our image-obsessed, patriarchal society. Anorexics and bulimics were merely mirroring cultural attitudes that encouraged women to use unnatural measures to subjugate their own physical appetites to a warped beauty ideal of prepubescent thinness.

Both Bruch's indictment of family and the feminist analysis sounded logical, but neither theory made sense when compared with eating disorders statistics. Although about half of American women *and men* are on a diet at any given time and virtually everyone is exposed to advertising, the lifetime rate of anorexia and bulimia nervosa combined is less than 7 percent of the U.S. population. This amounts to nearly twenty-one million people, without doubt a significant problem. Yet while the rate of anorexia has remained essentially unchanged since 1991, the rate of obesity has tripled, to include more than 30 percent of all Americans. So when I read Caroline Knapp's declaration in *Appetites* that all "white, affluent, and highly educated" women suffer from self-deprivation akin to anorexia, I was more than a little skeptical.

"How deprived," Knapp wondered, "how unentitled, how

full of sorrow and self-hatred did the essential self become?" The answer, in her experience as a former anorexic—and in mine—was too often too full. But recent surveys suggest that rates of anorexia nervosa throughout Asia and in nonwhite populations as far from Western culture as Curaçao and Ghana are about the same as they are in the Western world (though in societies such as Japan the stigma against seeking psychiatric treatment means that many cases go undiagnosed). Between 10 and 15 percent of anorexics and bulimics are men. And in 1994 *Essence* magazine surveyed two thousand women and concluded that the proportion of African-American women struggling with eating disorders matched the proportion of white women. Do their eating disorders get at the same "complicated questions" as white women's struggles with appetite? If not, why do these disparate individuals all engage in the same behavior? And *do* all white, affluent, educated women in fact feel compelled to deprive themselves?

I asked my friend Lindsay to read Knapp's work and tell me what she thought. Lindsay, a licensed therapist with three graduate degrees, is the mother of two teenage daughters. She, Knapp, and I were born just a few years apart, all in New England. Lindsay was a victim of incest as a child and later suffered from severe depression and post-traumatic stress disorder. She has hardly led a charmed life. Yet Lindsay flaunts her bodacious figure and vehemently rejects the suggestion that all white women in our culture are victims of fear and despair. A self-described feminist, she told me she was moved by Knapp's personal story, but her sympathy sprang from the fact that this experience "was so far from my own. Knapp's worldview, which she presented as a 'woman's' worldview, was not mine. As a woman who's never had an eating disorder, that annoyed me."

Tiffany Rush-Wilson's background bears little resemblance to Knapp's. Tiffany spent her early childhood in inner-city Cleveland, surrounded by her extended African-American family. Her family moved to middle-class Shaker Heights, a suburb of Cleveland, when Tiffany was thirteen. That year she "decided to be anorexic" by restricting her diet to McDonald's french fries, but it didn't take. Her parents refused to accept her argument that she needed to lose weight and insisted she eat normal meals with the family. A year later, she read an article in YM magazine about bulimia and followed it like an instruction manual. Tiffany powered her way through college and graduate school, took up marathon running, held down sometimes as many as five jobs at a time. No matter how much she achieved or earned, however, it never seemed enough. For eleven years she remained secretly bulimic. Every time she reached out for help, she was told she couldn't possibly have an eating disorder because black girls were "culturally protected." Now thirty-three, married with a daughter of her own and a Ph.D. in psychology, Tiffany specializes in the treatment of eating and body image disorders. She knows that cultural protection is a myth. "It's in me still," she said of bulimia. "Dormant, but I have to watch for it, especially when I get stressed."

University of New Mexico psychiatrist Joel Yager told me that his work in and around Albuquerque, with patients from rural as well as urban communities, has convinced him that eating disorders span all cultures. He recalled one patient who lived "a hundred miles from anywhere. Little town, father is a fifth-generation Hispanic maintenance worker for the county; the mother is a nurse in a residential home for retarded kids. This kid has been raised by these lovely blue-collar people, no competition at all in this family. She doesn't have to succeed to make them look good; it's not that kind of a family. But she's a born perfectionist. Not only is she the first kid in the family to go to college, but she had it in her mind when she was seven years old that she was going to college. That's her sense of self. So when her jerky narcissistic boyfriend went out with her best friend when she was fourteen years old, she started to think, maybe I'm too fat. She realized there was something weird about that, but it stuck in her mind. Eventually the girl became anorexic, just like one of her cousins—and one of her aunts."

A final example that throws Knapp's conception of eating disorders into question is my Santa Fe friend Carol. Duly white and affluent, Carol grew up with a mother who did everything in her power to suppress her three daughters' appetites. The girls were forbidden second helpings at the family table and allowed to speak only in order of seniority (being the youngest of three, Carol rarely opened her mouth). Mrs. York considered excess weight gain a punishable offense and, like Candace's mother, kept herself trim and her home immaculate. Yet Carol emerged from her childhood exuberant, with an appetite for love, food, and art that would not quit. In adulthood, this lust for life has buoyed her through her long battle with cancer. When I recently told her about another of our classmates who had slipped into anorexia after her son went off to college, Carol said, "Maybe it's because my health is so precious to me; I can't understand why anyone would purposely go hungry."

There were doubtless common reasons why Caroline Knapp, Tiffany Rush-Wilson, Candy Lunt, and I all developed eating disorders while Lindsay and Carol did not. There were doubtless related reasons why, long after recovering, Candace, Tiffany, and I still tended toward aggressive self-discipline and restraint. I was beginning to think these had as much to do with how we were wired as where, when, or how we were raised.

*   *   *

Kim Olensky at sixteen radiated the kind of wholesomeness one associates with Miss America. She dated the captain of the basketball team and had the votes to be queen of the prom before school even started. Toward the end of junior year, however, she began to lose weight. Over summer vacation she dropped thirty pounds. She traded her miniskirts for baggy jeans, and her boyfriend the jock for a poet. Senior year Kim carried a pillow because she lacked enough flesh to cushion her tailbone when she sat down. Speculation around school abounded. Something must have happened. Maybe to do with the basketball player. Maybe to do with her hard-drinking father. Maybe she just got fed up with the fawning of all those idiot boys. No one I knew ever got close enough to ask.

The last time I saw Kim, we had recently graduated from college and both happened to be visiting Carol, who then lived in New York. My weight was back to normal, but Kim still needed her pillow. The three of us spent an evening together talking about the older, wealthy men she and I were dating and Carol's recent breakup with her boyfriend from high school. Then, like Candy, Kim moved and left no forwarding address. We had no idea what had become of her until a quarter century later, when Carol's search for her "disappeareds" turned up a number for Kim's older sister.

Which was how I found myself standing outside the condominium complex in Santa Barbara, California, where Kim lives today. As the buzzer sounded to let me in, I thought hopefully of Candace—how much she now resembled herself as a healthy young child . . . but I never knew Kim as a little girl.

The door opened and we blinked at each other, straining for recognition. Kim was still petite. It was difficult to tell just how petite, since she wore several layers of black Polartec on this warm fall day, but the resemblance to her past self ended there. Her cheeks now were full, her face powdered and blushed, her hair cut short, fluffed, and colored a deep auburn. I would have passed her on the street without a glimmer of recognition, and I sensed she felt the same about me.

I had brought as a gift a block print from Carol of her New Mexico kitchen, but when we moved inside I held back. The picture was full of color and shape, bowls filled with shells, a bunch of flowers, two dogs, a cat, a rocking chair. Kim's condo was champagne white. We sat on an antique French empire settee. A cut-crystal light fixture hung above the polished dining table. Spotless as Candace's childhood home, the place felt more like a model apartment on the Upper East Side of Manhattan than the beachfront condo of a girl who once lived in overalls and Birkenstocks.

I considered the absence of pictures on the walls. Zero photographs—no family, no pets, no friends. "How long have you lived here?"

"Three years."

I decided to give Kim the print. "Thank you!" she said. But she hesitated before taking it and awkwardly set it down.

"What brought you to California?"

"Escape." Abruptly, she stood. "Let's get out of here."

We drove to a nearby coffee shop where Kim ordered tea— no sugar, no milk. "Anything else?" I eyed the display of glazed cookies and muffins. I wasn't hungry but would gladly have shared something. Kim shook her head.

She told me how she'd earned a graduate degree in sociology, then worked as a paralegal and later entered public relations. She built her own consulting business and eventually married a prominent corporate executive in Atlanta. He was ten years older and had three children. They were together for nearly fifteen years. Then she caught him in an affair with one of his clients.

I told Kim about the meltdown of my own marriage. We both had older husbands, and I, too, was a stepmother, though my stepson was now grown. "When we separated," I said, "it seemed as if everyone in the family went into hiding. For the first time in twenty years I felt alone. I immediately stopped eating."

Kim nodded. "I lost more weight before the divorce than I did in high school. It diverted attention from what was really going on. Oh, so *you're* the problem." Anorexia, she explained, offered a familiar haven where she was in full control and where her husband couldn't hurt her. It also visibly signaled that something was wrong which needed immediate attention. But Kim's husband refused to admit that he was contributing to her distress. Instead, he turned the signal back on her, making her the culprit. Not only did he claim her illness was the reason he'd strayed but he also used it as justification to end the marriage. And yet, she had to admit that the divorce and relapse had prompted her to resume long-term therapy, which she believed saved her life. She was now "up to" 105 and studying to become a clinical therapist herself.

Kim had been so ill in high school, I couldn't bear to imagine the damage she must have done to her body during this recent ordeal. I asked if her psychotherapeutic training had helped her understand why she returned to anorexia, specifically, as her retreat.

She turned her teacup between her palms. "You never met my family, did you?"

"I saw your mother a few times," I said. "Small, quiet, dressed in tweeds and sensible shoes."

"She managed a garden supply company." Kim rolled her eyes. "Even when we were little, there was never food in the house. I mean, there was food to cook, but no sandwich bread or fruit or crackers—you know, ready *fuel*. It didn't seem to occur to her that growing kids might need to eat more than she did."

I was confused. "You think *that's* why—?"

"Just an early indication. Both my parents drank too much." She shrugged. "I never could trust her to keep me safe."

Safety, it turned out, counted for a great deal because Kim's father became violent when drunk. But in talking about him, Kim was surprisingly generous. "He was a self-made man," she said. "As a child, after immigrating from Russia, he lived in a shed behind the boardinghouse his parents managed. That was how they survived the Depression." Eventually he earned a graduate degree and built a successful insurance firm. "But he never got over the shame of his childhood, the poverty. No matter how much he achieved—or how much attention he got—it was never enough." Many men of his generation and circumstances drank. But alcohol ignited Kim's father's rage. The more he drank, the more he punished his family. Breaking things. Yelling.

By junior year in high school, Kim wanted out. Her weight

loss wasn't just about changing her social identity. She wanted
to disappear. Christmas of senior year her older sister, Sarah,
came home, took one look at Kim, and shouted at her parents,
"What's the matter with you? Can't you see she's killing herself?" These were two excellent questions, which no one had
ever asked before. At Sarah's insistence, Kim's mother took her
to a psychotherapist.

"Intervention made a big difference," Kim recalled. "I felt
safe there to tell the truth." Unfortunately, just as her husband
would twenty years later, Kim's parents insisted she was "the
sick one." Neither would participate in therapy.

The showdown came at the beginning of summer just before
Kim graduated from high school. She'd invited a few close
friends from the literary magazine staff over to swim one night
around ten o'clock. Actually, they were skinny-dipping, but
they kept all the lights off. They didn't make much noise. Kim's
mother was asleep. Then her father came home. "He came to
the door and took one look at us, and I knew there was going
to be hell to pay. But he didn't say anything." Instead he went
back inside the house, and a minute later they heard a scream
from the master bedroom. By the time Kim and her friends got
upstairs her father had thrown her mother across the room. She
had curled into a fetal position against the wall to protect herself as he beat her, accusing her of raising a family of sluts. Kim
screamed at him to stop, but her father just bellowed back, "Get
those assholes out of here!"

She left then and never really returned. Neither parent ever
acknowledged what had happened. Kim became inseparable
from the friends who had been with her that night. They went
off to college together. Her weight, though far too low, stabilized,
and eventually she quit therapy.

Then she married a self-made older man who sounded suspi-
ciously like her father. "We never stop trying to make our childhood right," she said.

Perhaps, I thought, but Kim's older sister seemed to have

managed. And I assumed the point of treatment was to find a way to do the same.

I asked Kim if she was dating anyone now. She pushed the thought away. "My life is very quiet. I work at the clinic. I attend classes. I read a lot and see my sister occasionally. This"— she gestured to indicate my visit—"is a big deal." Her smile held a challenge. No self-pity allowed, she seemed to be saying. No regrets. And, above all, no self-indulgence.

I shivered, envying Kim her Polartec. The afternoon had turned brisk. "Will you call again?" she asked as we got up to leave. I took this as an invitation and promised I would, but when I phoned a few weeks later she wasn't home. I left a message but got no response. Twice more I tried. At Christmas I sent a card. No answer.

In *The Noonday Demon* Andrew Solomon writes, "Depression is a response to past loss, and anxiety is a response to future loss," but the two states often feel inseparable. One reason, he suggests, is that depression and anxiety share a single set of genes. These happen to lie close to the genes for alcoholism. All three of these genetic hammers seemed to have slammed Kim's family, and she was still fighting the reverberations. Yet out of four siblings, only she had responded by physically shrinking herself. As I tried to make sense of this I kept coming back to Kim's use of words like *escape* and *safe*, her social isolation, the careful blankness of her condo—as if she didn't dare commit to making a home for herself, even after three years.

Anxiety is a primal instinct in all of us and a basic necessity for survival. Fear prompts us to freeze before the grizzly notices us strolling down the trail, to flee that car rolling toward us before it gets too close, and to fight the kitchen fire that threatens our home. But more than two thirds of anorexics and bulimics have a lifelong history of anxiety disorders: they get stuck in either the freeze, flight, or fight mode, even when not under any actual threat. Some feel an overwhelming need to withdraw from society; some seize with panic at the slightest criticism; some become so tense they lash out at their best friends. Many never feel safe enough to relax yet find in eating disorders a perverse mode of escape.

Here's how this escape works: you flee anxiety by pulling into yourself; you purge your fear by vomiting it up; you become so obsessive about your body that nothing else in the world seems to matter. The result is that you feel you have this body—your contained world—under control. So while a different woman in Kim's position might have called the police on her father or cleaned out her husband's bank account and taken a lover herself, Kim instead exerted maximum control over her physical self.

What, then, determines how we manage anxiety? This question, it seemed to me, could be central to understanding not only who "gets" eating disorders in the first place but who successfully recovers—and how. For answers, I turned to Michael Strober, director of the Eating Disorder Program at UCLA's Neuropsychiatric Institute.

Now in his late fifties, Strober has treated eating disorders for more than thirty years. He has a global reputation as editor of the *International Journal of Eating Disorders* and, with his ink-brush eyebrows and barely audible voice, gives a somewhat daunting first impression. So as we sat in the cafeteria below his office, I tried to sound as if I knew what I was asking. "It seems to me," I fumbled, "that many of my lifelong habits—compulsive exercising, biting my nails, habitually apologizing for myself—may be related to my having been anorexic."

During the pause that followed, I was afraid Strober was going to dismiss me outright. Instead, he blew my suspicion wide open. "There's minimal cultural influence in anorexia nervosa," he said flatly. "It's not causal. It only contributes if the inherent risk is there."

Cultural influence, I assumed, meant the usual culprits: *Shape* magazine, weight-conscious parents, size-2 celebrities, and school yard fat jokes. But what exactly did he mean by inherent risk?

Strober reeled off a list of typical anorexic qualities: "perfectionistic, cautious, highly regimented, and disciplined; and they suffer from inadequacy that is entirely self-perceived. These traits are largely inherent—not exclusively so, but it's well documented that anorexia nervosa has the strongest correlation to temperament of any psychological illness. Bulimia nervosa also has a correlation but less so."

This was research speak. I needed plain English. "Inherent," I repeated. "Are we talking DNA?"

"Our research suggests that anorexia has a strong genetic component. Yes." Since 1996 Strober had been working with a multinational team, led by Dr. Walter Kaye at the University of Pittsburgh School of Medicine, to search for possible genetic links. By analyzing genetic samples from across the United States, Canada, England, and Germany, they so far had identified "susceptibility genes" for restricting anorexia nervosa on chromosome 1, and for bulimia on chromosome 10. Strober told me that identical twins of anorexic subjects have a 50 to 60 percent likelihood of developing the eating disorder, even if raised apart, whereas fraternal twins of anorexics have the same 14 percent risk that their other siblings have. Girls in families with no history of eating disorders, meanwhile, run less than a 3 percent chance of becoming anorexic.

I thought of my own family. I mentioned that several of my nieces had struggled with bulimia.

"Not surprising," Strober said. He'd found that immediate family members of anorexics were twelve times more likely to develop anorexia than people without a family history of the disorder, but they were also four times more likely to suffer from bulimia. "What's interesting about these results is that they suggest several different eating disorders may link to a common genetic source." Compulsive overeating and binge eating disorder may also have genetic roots. Prader-Willi syndrome, for example, is a chromosomal disorder, affecting both sexes, that causes an insatiable appetite for food, beginning in early childhood. However, Strober cautioned, the temperamental and physical profiles of compulsive and binge eaters tend to be much more varied and variable than the profiles of individuals with anorexia and bulimia. Overeaters are nearly as likely to be male as female and may be overweight or of normal weight, which suggests that genes play a less consistent role than they appear to in anorexia and bulimia.

The latest research did, however, point to links between anorexia nervosa and obsessive-compulsive behavior, anxiety disorders, and depression—all of which tend to persist long after the eating disorder. At UCLA, Strober said, anorexic and bulimic patients are considered recovered when they maintain a healthy weight and no longer obsessively count calories, binge or purge or manically exercise; yet even years later these recovered patients will show abnormally high rates of anxiety and obsessive thinking, especially perfectionism. "The solution is not to eliminate these traits but to learn to manage them. So in treatment we try to move patients to a new framework, to enable them to accept growth and change." The problem is that growing and changing run directly counter to the craving for order and familiarity that typifies anorexia nervosa. Carefully constructed rituals and disciplines protect an illusion of emotional safety. By challenging those rigid patterns of behavior and thinking, treatment threatens to expose "unacceptable" emotions like fear and grief and despair. "That's why anorexia nervosa in particular is so difficult to treat and why there are some patients who will never get well. Bulimic individuals, while also typically perfectionistic, are less restrained and more impulsive. And they generally respond better to treatment."

I pictured a scale of temperament with extremely compulsive restricting anorexics at one end and extremely impulsive bulimics at the other. "Do some recover, then, only to shift that rigidity—or impulsivity—to anxiety-reducing habits that have nothing to do with food?"

"It's possible."

Connect the dots. I asked Strober one last key question: "Has anyone studied the daily lives of people who've *recovered* from eating disorders?"

"Outcome studies. Rates of recovery, suicide, relapse—that sort of thing, but not much on subjective experience. Work, marriage, parenting styles. Is that what you mean?"

I nodded.

"It's a wide-open field." He smiled and extended his hand. "Let me know what you find out."

If Strober was right, then much of the blame that had long surrounded eating disorders—and that shaped my own assumptions in *Solitaire*—was misplaced. Perhaps no single factor was at fault. Perhaps the impulse to blame, in fact, diverted essential energy and attention from the real business of recovery. Mothers who subscribed to *Vogue* might play a hand in some cases of anorexia, but according to Strober they no more "caused" the problem than chilly temperatures caused pneumonia. Nor did anorexics "choose" this infuriating and dangerous behavior—any more than they could snap out of their genetics on command.

To escape an obsession, I'd wanted to believe when writing *Solitaire*, one had only to recognize its pointlessness, and I had done that. But more than two decades later I realized that recovery was in many ways more complicated than the eating disorder itself. To make sense of it in my own life, I needed to go back to the turning point of my illness and this time search for the truth.

2

PORTRAIT OF A HUNGER ARTIST

The Face of Fear

> Just try to explain to anyone the art of fasting!
> Anyone who has no feeling for it cannot be
> made to understand it.
> —Franz Kafka, *A Hunger Artist*

THE SUMMER OF 1973 was a time when most of my Yale class-mates were chasing opportunities—to intern at CBS or study at the Sorbonne, trek in Nepal or go lobster fishing in Maine. I instead chose to spend the summer after my sophomore year alone in New Haven losing weight. By night, I house-sat for the chair of the music department. Mornings, I matted prints at the Yale Art Gallery. Afternoons and weekends, I retreated to the otherwise vacant undergraduate painting studio and worked obsessively on self-portraits. My primary food source was a ten-pound bag of oranges, which lasted me six weeks. My primary source of inspiration was a collection of mirrors in varying sizes, which I positioned around my easel. Though the paradox was lost on me then, it dumbfounds me today: as if playing hide-and-seek with myself, I fasted to minimize my body even as I painted canvas after canvas featuring this body as a centerpiece.

I *was* hiding and seeking myself that summer, but the game was more of a psychological search-and-destroy mission than child's play. I worked from a mirror tilting upward, so the reflected image peered down her nose. I imagined this external reflection berating my hidden, internal self: "You are nothing. You are weak, pathetic. Just you try to match *my* power and complexity." The tyrant I saw in that mirror had ruled me since I was fourteen years old. Part of me, yet apart from me, she despised me. She warned me not to eat, berated me for feeling hunger, ridiculed my loneliness. The only way to avoid a life of utter failure was to do exactly as she said.

Of course, we all are prisoners of our conscience, to varying degrees. Philosophers dating back to Plato have assigned the intellect the right and duty to rule over physical appetites. Aristotle believed this management to be essential for the creation of a harmonious sense of self. For people with eating disorders, however, this management escalates into an internal war, with the body as battleground. That summer, my tyrannical conscience was winning the war. Her haughty expression dominated each portrait, sneering or simply staring in cold indifference. In only one of the dozen or so paintings I produced in those months did her fearful captive venture an appearance.

I began that interior with broad, easy strokes to catch the fluorescent shimmer of heat, the bald planes of the walls and door, the hard angles of empty stretchers, the vacancy of the studio. As I zeroed in on the mirror propped in the left-hand corner, I added turpentine to thin the medium, used progressively softer, finer brushes, and worked long into the night. The figure in the mirror started rough, sketchy, and large, but day after day her reflection kept shrinking. The more she shrank, the more compulsively and minutely I worked at her, and yet somehow, the more precisely I painted her, the more indefinite she grew. Studying the finished canvas thirty years later I am struck by the reflection's disembodiment. Her face resembles a miniature mask, eyes pocketed in shadow, the mouth a thin flat line. She looks out, as if trapped, from her mirror cage within that blazing room. "Dare," she seems to say to anyone who will pay attention. "Step through this looking glass and tear off this mask. Find out what lies underneath."

My weight dropped below 90 pounds that summer. I supplemented my oranges with chocolate chips—all of six a day, which I furtively dug from the undersides of cookies stocked in the art gallery kitchenette (no rule but my own prohibited me from eating the cookies whole and by the fistful). Back at the house where I was staying, the refrigerator was full of Tupperware containers the professor's wife had left for me with helpings of stroganoff, pudding, macaroni, but I left this fattening comfort food to mold. When ravenous, I would break the seal on one of the mason jars in the pantry and steal a single teaspoonful of homemade plum or blackberry jam. As I sneaked each taste, I assured myself that my hosts (who had told me they didn't care what I ate) would think I took nothing. In my invented world that summer, consumption constituted a crime.

As that July ebbed into August, real crimes in Vietnam and the Watergate hearings filled the airwaves, but I didn't turn on the television. I never looked at a newspaper, rarely even listened to music. I'd broken up with my boyfriend that spring, had no friends in town, and would not let myself even make a phone call. I often went entire days without speaking—unable to get a word in over my inner taskmaster, who never shut up: "You fat, disgusting slob, you'll never be thin enough, good enough, smart enough, tough or talented enough. . . ." When my mother phoned to check on me, I refused her offers to visit as well as her exhortations for me to come home. "I'm fine," I insisted. "I'm getting a lot of painting done. Just leave me alone." Reluctantly, she backed off. I needed to prove my independence. She knew that. I knew that. But prove it to whom?

This was one question I didn't dare ask as I put in my hours working alone in the gallery's conservation department, then at the studio painting as long as I could stand it. Finally I'd walk miles to the house I was tending and fall, ravenous, into sleep.

Late one August afternoon, I was halfway across campus when I noticed footsteps echoing off the stone walls of Commons. They sounded so loud that I stopped, but no one else was there. The sky was cloudless, Magritte bright; and beneath it, the quad stretched, silent now. Berkeley and Calhoun, like all Yale's dorms, were locked up for the summer, and Sterling and Beinecke libraries had closed for the night. The day's heat had withered the lawn. Nothing moved. Not a car. Not a leaf. Even New Haven's usual rumble of distant construction had ceased. As the thick air pressed and held me, the silence seemed to grow into a roar. It was as if the entire city had emptied.

My head began to pound. The weight of it doubled me over. I was seized by a dizziness, hard and pitiless as a hunger pang. I thought of all the people I'd spent years pushing away: friends, parents, my boyfriend, teachers. Just leave me alone, I'd pleaded. One by one, they'd all obeyed; and now, finally, I had exactly what I'd claimed I wanted: nothing. For the first time, it dawned on me just how little nothing really matters, how little *I* would matter if I continued to isolate and minimize myself. What was I so *afraid* of? I had no idea.

I lifted my head. A moving truck sped down College Street, its accelerator gunning. I pushed myself forward. Through the diesel wake poured a stream of music—piano, some experimental dissonance out of Stoeckel Hall, and I thought with a surprise of longing of the Scott Joplin ragtime records I'd noticed but never played in the house where I was staying. What was it that held me back? Nothing.

I turned the corner onto Prospect Avenue. At the beginning of the summer, standing on this corner, my roommate Patty had suggested that I take the train to visit her in Boston. I'd told her no, I'd be too busy, but she persisted. We'd have fun, she said.

We'd play. She'd show me were she lived and introduce me to her friends. All I had to do was call, and she would pick me up.

I would go, I decided, walking faster. I would call and Patty would collect me in her battered red VW. I'd see the beachfront restaurant where she wore a silly Martha Washington uniform and served her customers popovers. She'd take me out in her sloop around the point of Marblehead. We'd visit her friend Jay in Cambridge and have dinner at the Harvest. And I would quit pretending that hunger was artistic or ennobling or good. Hunger, I finally had to admit, was wasting my life.

I listened to Scott Joplin that night. I went to Boston that weekend. I willed myself to follow Patty's example and began, tentatively, to increase the amount I allowed myself to eat. But three years later, as I wrote *Solitaire*, I was still trying to puzzle out what had happened that August afternoon. Unable to make sense of what had actually occurred, I altered the moment for effect in my memoir, turning it into an upbeat ending. I characterized my state of mind not as a meltdown but as "elation and freedom." I claimed I'd felt "pure delight in just looking and standing still." I wanted to strike an uplifting note on which to decisively conclude my adolescent ordeal.

But a turning point, while critical, is not the same as a conclusion. That shock of silence on the quad was simply the moment when, in psychologist Sheila Reindl's words, I sensed that I'd reached my "limit of distress." Virtually everyone who recovers from an eating disorder experiences such a moment. It might take a comment, a look, or the scare of a medical prognosis, but suddenly the obsession that just seconds before seemed all-powerful is revealed, like the Wizard of Oz, to be nothing more than the trick of a frightened mind. Once this truth is revealed it becomes safe to say, "I'm sick of this," or simply, "Enough!"

Karen Armstrong, whose memoir *The Spiral Staircase* describes her passage through anorexia following seven years as a nun, wrote of her turning point, after three hospitalizations, as a sensory epiphany. "The color, vibrancy, and sheer energy of the outside world greeted me like a gift. Food tasted better, the air smelled sweeter, and ordinary little privacies seemed the greatest of privileges. . . . I started to eat normally again, quite spontaneously. . . . That phase was over." But Armstrong's reference to her "anorexic phase" is, I think, telling. She had taken an important step forward by recovering the will to eat, yet she was still a long way from recovering the true fullness of her life. "The new joy demanded effort," she acknowledged. "It would be a lifelong task, requiring alert attention."

Patterns of eating, thinking, feeling, and behaving that have taken years to develop and that may stem from inborn disposition are not going to reverse in a single afternoon. I know this now from my own experience. I also know it from Caroline Knapp, who at forty-one wrote, "I'm still prone to periods of isolation, still more fearful of the world out there and more averse to pleasure and risk than I'd like to be; I still direct more energy toward controlling and minimizing appetites than toward indulging them; I am one of the least spontaneous people I know." I know it from Marya Hornbacher's observation following her long battle with bulimia: "Always, there is an odd distance between you and the people you love and the people you meet, a barrier, thin as the glass of a mirror." I also know it from Jessica Mason, a twenty-five-year old Australian who reached her turning point at eighteen, yet still is in anorexia's grip.

Jessica's father, Trevor, had no illusions when he e-mailed me from Sydney in 2004. While searching online for resources that might help Jessica, he had come across my Web site and my appeal for interview subjects. Despite extensive treatment, he told me, Jessica remained underweight, obsessed with dieting, and deeply depressed. Trevor thought her story might interest me. He also was grasping at the chance that I, as someone who had recovered, might offer her new insight, suggestions, or hope.

The Mason family was in entertainment: Trevor a television producer in Sydney and his wife, Emma, a theater set designer.

Jessica, their only child, Trevor wrote, was "an outstanding actor, designer, presenter, communicator. As a child and teenager she seemed destined to go far. She went to drama school, and all went wrong. An intimidating tutor and anorexia combined to tell her she was no good. She left. Tragedy really. She has more recently worked as a tutor in television and film courses that I run, and she is loved by her students. She refuses to see her talent. As designer for this country's major youth fashion contest, also run by us, she has been outstanding. Again she believes not." I had to smile, though, when he followed this with the abashed admission that his wife, who knew the therapeutic drill, was reading over his shoulder and "reckons the above shrieks parental expectations and ignores the point that Jessica is a stunning young woman with loads of personality, and to be honest we don't give a toss if she never acts again." These two seemed as proud of their daughter as they were desperate to help her.

I didn't want to give false hope, but I told the Masons I'd be pleased to include Jessica's story in my book and offer what wisdom I could. The one condition I set was that Jessica get in touch with me herself, of her own free choice. It seemed to me a positive sign that, when Jessica did write, she offered rather than requested help: "If I recover I am determined to extract something positive from this horrible illness and use my experience to assist others in some way. If I could start in a small manner now it would make me feel a little more valuable and give me something to think about other than food, exercise, and how disgusting I feel."

A week later, we spoke by phone. Jessica was living in Scarsdale, New York, with a friend from her last treatment center. She was learning to drive, trying to develop a sense of her own independence. She had a light, hesitant voice, and I pictured her as pale and fragile, nervously twisting the telephone cord as we talked. She and her friend had just come home from an evening in Manhattan seeing *The Good Body*, Eve Ensler's one-woman show. Like Ensler's earlier work *The Vagina Monologues*, this new show sounded a feminist alarm over the dismissal, betrayal, and denigration of the female body by Western culture. Ensler, a radical feminist for nearly thirty years, confessed onstage that her stomach "has become my tormentor, my distractor; it's my most serious committed relationship."

Jessica told me she found the performance insulting. "I thought it would be affirming of her healthy self," she said, "but the audience was laughing. And I was sitting there thinking, I do this, I think this, this is my life and people are laughing at it. I felt like they were trivializing it. Ensler has this forum and she was just skimming the surface. We know all this body-image stuff. What do we *do* about it?"

She told me her aunt, to whom she was close, was another fierce feminist, while her mother "was just very balanced. She never gave me one message or another. She was often on diets, but it was never a huge deal." Jessica's motivation to lose weight came not from her family but her peers. "I was teased mercilessly." Even today she has to fight the urge to go home and seek out the classmates who used to torment her for being chubby, just to hear them say, "My God, look how thin she is!"

The pressure to be thin was so intense and pervasive that *The Best Little Girl in the World*, a book written by psychiatrist Steven Levenkron to help anorexics, instead became Jessica's undoing. She and her friends thought of the book's anorexic character, Kessa, as "perfect." Far from being repulsed by Kessa's self-destructive rituals, the girls imitated them. Like the teens who today defiantly create "pro-ana" and "pro-mia" websites in *defense* of their "right" to have eating disorders, Jessica and her friends were so fixated on losing weight that they failed to notice the character was also losing her health, friends, beauty, and very nearly her life as she "succeeded" in minimizing her body. The fact that Kessa was shrinking herself onto a psychiatric ward never even registered. "So many of the girls I know read that book," Jessica told me, "my mum got it banned from the school library." But not in time. Jessica was diagnosed with anorexia at eleven, by which point, although she saw a doctor and knew what she was doing wasn't healthy, the terror of gaining weight ruled her. "I never ate three meals a day. Sometimes I was throwing up or taking laxatives or fasting." The only thing that gave her pleasure was the stage. "I knew I had to maintain some health to be able to act, so my passion for acting was kind of a godsend, really." She couldn't remember a time when she wasn't dancing or acting. "My mum was always reading and singing to me. I guess I decided I wanted to start auditioning for plays. When I was eleven I got the role of Scout in *To Kill a Mockingbird*. After that I was going to be an actor, and nothing was going to stop me."

I guess I decided I wanted. I was struck by the uncertainty of Jessica's recollection. And yet there was no doubt about the effect of that first starring role, that validation: *I am seen.* It reminded me of the day Wilhelmina accepted me into her modeling agency. I was fifteen. I was thrilled. After the meeting, when I sat down to lunch with my parents at a nearby restaurant, I didn't even want to eat. What I understand now is that excitement, physiologically, is anxiety's pleasurable twin. Both states can cause loss of appetite, trembling, dizziness, blushing, and rapid heartbeat. One feels good, the other bad, but both involve a highly volatile mix of hope and fear.

Jessica continued, "I had to get to the theater at least an hour before everyone else, so I was getting there two hours before the show. Before I could go onstage, I had to read the script through a certain number of times and ways. When I was in my first year of drama school and the anorexia started coming back, I had all these crystals around my makeup area. I had to focus on them for a certain amount of time and if something broke my concentration I'd take it as bad luck. I also had all these particular voice exercises and physical warm-ups. I wasn't sleeping at all, and I'd be sitting at the makeup table crying." Only onstage did Jessica pull herself together. There she could move outside of herself, into the role, the character. She always managed to perform for her audience. But then "I'd come off and be a mess again."

The obsessions wove together, making it more and more difficult for her to separate her eating disorder from her emotions and acting career. Her acting coach came to represent her inner tormentor. "Everything he said to me is stuff anorexia says to me: 'You're not trying hard enough, you're not honest enough, not good enough.'" Oddly, this coach was the one who forced Jessica to get help, if in a typically bullying fashion. She'd been in classes with him all day, hadn't eaten, and was exhausted as he went around the room, calling on each person for a dramatic response. "My brain wasn't functioning at all. He got to me and I just didn't care anymore. He said, 'I don't know what's going on with you, but whatever it is, you need to sort it out.' And he went on to the next person."

That was Jessica's turning point. She walked out of class and never went back. But her coach's anger won't let go of her, even years later. "I have recurring dreams about people in my life turning against me, giving up on me, or deciding I'm a selfish person. At the treatment center, I tried to leave one night because I thought they all hated me. Tiny things that weren't even meant as criticism had built up. The guard had to stop me running out the door."

One of the exercises in her group therapy sessions was to make a family tree and pinpoint anyone who'd had alcoholism, drug addiction, depression, anxiety or panic attacks, OCD, eating disorders. Everyone in the group, Jessica said, had family histories riddled with these disorders. "My own mother was very overanxious. There was always something dangerous around. 'Don't touch that, it's poisonous.' My grandmother was like that, too, and my great-aunt was anorexic. There's a lot of depression in my family and bits and pieces of alcoholism."

Jessica believes she has inherited a temperament that makes her feel unsafe in the world. Yet the world that most stridently reinforces her anxiety is precisely the one toward which she gravitates: Hollywood, glamour magazines, fashion. "I was obsessed with magazines. Anorexia was telling me I wasn't intelligent enough to read books. I couldn't understand them, I couldn't concentrate, I wouldn't retain any information. But you can always read magazines, and I was producing fashion shows at the time, so magazines were in the industry." Jessica fixated on Cameron Diaz. Her two best friends didn't even know who Cameron Diaz was. They told Jessica magazines like *Us* and *InStyle* were "a load of crap. They said, 'Why would we waste our money on magazines? Much rather buy a book. The photos are all doctored. Why bother?' "

Jessica couldn't believe it. "You don't want to look like Cameron Diaz?"

Her friend answered, "Maybe I shouldn't have had that bag of chips because it's not healthy, but Cameron Diaz's body doesn't occur to me."

Jessica thought, *I am brainwashed.*

It would be reassuring if that epiphany had turned her life around. But she obsessed about those magazines the same way she obsessed about exercise and weight loss. She couldn't bring herself to quit until she reached the "safety" of her California treatment center, where personality and fashion magazines were banned. When Jessica spoke about this program her voice turned wan. In Australia she'd seen psychologists, internists, homeopaths, nutritionists, anyone she and her parents could find who might be able to help her, but nothing had broken the hold of anorexia. Finally, she'd decided the only solution was to go into a residential facility that specialized in eating disorders. "I needed to be in a place where I couldn't do any of the things I was doing and all my power was taken away. Which is not what happened, but that's how I felt."

Jessica's therapist recommended a program in a quiet neighborhood north of Los Angeles. There were courtyard fountains and wind chimes outside her bedroom window. For four months the voice in her head backed off. She talked and listened in therapy. She allowed herself to play. She filled coloring books with hot pinks and deep blues. She exercised horses, painted, made collages and jewelry. "I felt for the first time in years I had all this room to be creative." But her weight remained low—too low for antidepressants to do much for her—and her parents didn't have the resources to keep her in the program indefinitely (few insurance plans inside or outside the United States pay for long-term treatment of eating disorders). In New York, even though her assignment was to stay in therapy and gain weight, her compulsiveness returned. Now she stacked her days with Pilates, yoga, the gym, walking, breakfast, lunch, dinner, three snacks, plus sessions with her therapist and nutritionist and time to write in her journal. "So many things take up so much space, and the obsessive thoughts are getting worse and worse the more hopeless I feel."

As for planning life on her own, "I can hardly concentrate on an e-mail. I feel like it would be irresponsible of me to even drive a car. Power scares me. What if I did something wrong? I couldn't be relied on, I might fall apart." The California treatment program itself had become an obsession. It was the one place on the planet where Jessica felt she could get better. "I'm desperate to get back there because I need to feel safe enough to let some of this not be my responsibility."

As we concluded our conversation, I could sense just how frustrated Jessica's parents must be, how frustrated my own parents must once have been watching me defiantly, persistently waste my body and life. Jessica had received the kind of therapy I'd long believed could have spared me my anorexic ordeal, yet she remained a prisoner of her obsessions into her mid-twenties—the age I was when writing *Solitaire*.

"My belief," psychiatrist Mark Warren told me, "is that the perceived threat is ultimate destruction." Warren, who is currently medical director of the Cleveland Center for Eating Disorders, based this remark not specifically on Jessica but on hundreds of patients—women and men of all ages, backgrounds, and ethnicities—that he has treated over twenty years. "The real underlying fear is that the self will dissolve and one will cease to exist. I think only fear that profound would produce symptoms this profound."

Recovery, then, would mean cultivating the faith that those fears will not come true. "There's a Westernized notion of self that's not accurate," Warren explained. "It says there's a self trapped inside this meat I call my body, which is different from the body, yet mirrored by it. So at some core level the anorexic believes that if she eats she'll become fat; and if her body is fat, her self must be disgusting and awful." Warren's view of the self is more interactive. "I think it really is this constantly created experience that happens at the boundary between the person and the environment. 'Who I am' is constantly being mediated by my internal experience and my external experience." He tries to help recovering patients "come to the surface" enough to fully sense—through tasting, touching, smelling, and hearing, as well as seeing—the world around them. They learn to trust that the world, including their family and friends, will not hurt them. Gradually they discover that the world can be a source of support and satisfaction rather than fear.

People with eating disorders tend to resist this notion, Warren said, because, in their experience, the external world is a danger zone. "Certain temperaments respond to anxiety by pulling inward. Their instincts tell them, 'Don't go out to meet the world—you'll have a panic attack and it will be horrible for you. Inside is where the safety is.' " That message, reinforced through experiences as commonplace as school yard name-calling or a bullying drama coach—or as violent as an alcoholic father—can fuel the kind of changes to one's anatomy and brain chemistry that Peter Kramer, in Listening to Prozac, describes as encoded memory. This coding, Kramer says, can raise one's baseline sensitivity so that it takes progressively less and less stress to trigger feelings of anxiety. Eventually, you're in a constant state of high alert.

If this theory is correct, then the temperaments that are prone to anxiety should be the same temperaments that are prone to eating disorders. In 2001 Boston University psychologists Drew Westen and Jennifer Harnden-Fischer published a study that bore this out. People who develop anorexia and bulimia, they found, tend to fall into three distinct—and mostly lifelong—temperamental groups, all marked by high anxiety.

The first group, which the study labeled *overcontrolled*, includes most restricting anorexics and a minority of bulimics. They "feel like they have nothing inside." They avoid social contact; tightly control their appetites for food and for sex; limit their pleasures; and withdraw from excitement, sensation, and risk. Think of Kim Olensky in her silent white condo, Jessica Mason's desperation to feel safe, and Caroline Knapp's fear of "the world out there."

The second, or *perfectionistic*, group includes most bulimics and a minority of restricting anorexics. These are the conscientious "good girls" who aim to please, excel, and conform. They worry about the details but are often so fearful of making a mistake that they can't get their work in on time. They read an arched eyebrow as contempt, a frown as a stiletto through the heart. They are intensely self-critical. This description catapulted me back to Carol's kitchen: Candace Lunt's meticulous fishes and my own artistic paralysis.

The third, or *undercontrolled*, group is split about evenly between bulimics and anorexics who binge and purge. "Their emotions are intense, their behaviors are impulsive, they tend to fly into rages instead of expressing their anger passively or turning it inward, and they desperately seek relationships to soothe themselves." Like human metronomes, this group might start a diet because their boyfriends tease them, succumb to a billboard's temptation by stealing a Big Mac, then purge after seeing a magazine article about how much Mary-Kate Olsen weighs. This erratic portrait fits Marya Hornbacher, who wrote in *Wasted* about her substance abuse, sexual promiscuity, and bulimia. Like many in this group, she also cut. "After my eating disorder was 'over,' " she recalled, "I would go in blind search for something else with which to tear myself apart. I found a razor blade worked quite well. . . . Carving away at the body to—symbolically and literally—carve up an imperfect soul."

There is a degree of crossover, particularly between the perfectionists and the undercontrolled group, and particularly during recovery. About half of all restricting anorexics pass, as I did, through a stage of bulimia on their way to normal weight. In my case, I reached a point where I felt desperate to escape my tense little good-girl persona. So I dabbled in drugs. I started and quit jobs on a whim. I asked a friend of a friend to lend me five thousand dollars, which I had no way of repaying—a request that would have mortified me a year earlier and that makes me cringe today. Such an extreme and temporary shift in behavior makes sense if you think of bulimia as a signal of surrender. When the rigidity and compulsiveness of anorexia give way, the pendulum of appetite swings wildly for a time. Take in, expel. Stuff, empty. Sate, deny. Experiment, suppress. These are the dueling messages of bulimia. How do we know when we have eaten enough? When we have enough attention? Enough trophies or job offers, money or sex? Enough love? The all-or-nothing mind-set makes these questions perilous, and that mind-set is intrinsic to all eating disorders. That mind-set must change for the pendulum to reach a slower and healthier setting.

The Westen and Harnden-Fischer findings confirmed my suspicion that my own history of eating disorders could reveal some essential truths about my personality and my life. I didn't fully appreciate the scope of the findings, however, until I extended my interviews and realized that, whether I was talking to women or men, gays or straights, virtually everyone with a history of anorexia or bulimia seemed to fit one of these three personality categories. I also found that these descriptions rarely fit my friends who'd never had an eating disorder. It was as if the scientists had discovered that all anorexics had dyslexia or that bulimics were prone to traffic accidents. The ramifications extended far beyond eating and weight. As the study's authors wrote of the overcontrolled group, "If their attitudes toward their needs and feelings in general (and not just toward food) do not become the object of therapeutic attention, they are likely to change with treatment from being starving, unhappy, isolated, and emotionally constricted people to being relatively well fed, unhappy, isolated, and emotionally constricted people."

The question that must precede any meaningful or lasting change is, *Who cares?* Who cares whether you live or die, become a janitor or a rocket scientist, wear a size 2—or 20? The answer may seem obvious. Given the obsessiveness with which the eating disordered worry about their bodies, they clearly care a great deal. Just consider the language of these disorders. Though filled with *self-loathing*, anorexics excel at *self-discipline* and *selfless* acts of humility and generosity, which they often take to extremes of *self-denial* and *self-punishment*. Bulimics tend to be more *selfish* and *self-motivated*, but like anorexics, they are acutely *self-conscious* and riven with *self-doubt* and *self-contempt*. Both groups resist *self-awareness* even as they behave in ways that appear utterly *self-involved*. Eating disorders are all about the self—a self that somehow claims the center of attention while refusing to claim its own true needs and wants. Recovery begs the larger question: *If I'm the one who cares so much, who, then, am I?* Until we gain the courage to solve this complex riddle, the figure in the mirror—at any weight—will go right on tormenting us.

3

THE LAWS OF PERFECTION
Obsession and Compulsion

I would try to be perfect. It was safer there.
—Jane Fonda, *My Life So Far*

VANESSA QUINTERO BEGAN PREPARING for her book group meeting a week in advance. She made a pan of her signature rum fudge. On her way home from the office, she picked up several bottles of the group's favorite New Zealand chardonnay. She vacuumed her two-bedroom house from front to back, polished her mother's silver, hand-washed her grandmother's crystal glasses and serving bowls. On the day of the meeting she shopped at the neighborhood farmers' market for fresh romaine and heirloom tomatoes, and at a nearby Swiss bakery for baguettes. When she got home she poached chicken and salmon, peeled kiwis, folded starched white napkins into bread baskets, filled the living room with bouquets of blue irises, which matched the floral wallpaper, rearranged the furniture, took a quick shower, applied a fresh coat of makeup, and changed into a pressed linen pantsuit that she hoped didn't make her look too matronly—Vanessa was fifty-seven and had recently gained two pounds. She almost had everything under control when I, a newcomer to the group, arrived fifteen minutes earlier than the other ten members. Vanessa welcomed me in with a fresh burst of activity, offering me a drink, filling silver bowls with nuts, fanning slivers of lemon and lime onto saucers, and calling to her husband, John, to decant the wine and brew the coffee but make sure he used the Peruvian decaf.

I stood before Vanessa's gleaming buffet table. "Can I help?"

"I don't know." She was breathing hard as she plucked at the edible pansies that garnished her presentation of chicken salad. "They don't look right. Can you help me fix them?"

Vanessa was a complete stranger, yet I felt I knew her inside out. This familiarity made me intensely curious. It also emboldened me. I told Vanessa the theme of this book. Then I plunged in: "Please don't take this the wrong way, but were *you* by chance ever anorexic?"

Her hand with its unruly pansy halted in midair. "How did you know!"

I touched her shoulder, laughing. "Because I behave exactly the same way."

"It's a source of control" was how another former anorexic described her perfectionism. "You feel like if the closet is arranged, then something in life is orderly. My relationships might not be, but this is something I have control over. It's the same thing as anorexia. It is all consuming."

Perfectionism is the single most consistent trait among both anorexics and bulimics. Most people who have had an eating disorder believe down to their nerve endings that perfection is a real, attainable noble state and that it is their right and duty to claim it, whether they are performing in a play, organizing a closet, planning a party, or anticipating a date. They probably can't tell you why they feel this way, but the ultimate standard nevertheless shadows them like a malevolent conscience.

The problem with perfection is that, by definition, it is unattainable, so perfectionists live in a state of perpetual frustration and disappointment. Just as Vanessa would never accept her edible pansies' arrangement as pretty enough, people with active anorexia and bulimia never feel that they are thin enough. Pressure from parents and peers and a culture that commands us to want more and better of everything from soft drinks to sports cars surely doesn't help, but the true root of this dissatisfaction is internal. Perfectionism, like shyness, obstinacy, curiosity, and impulsiveness, is a function of the temperament one is born with.

I did not always believe this. I used to think perfectionism was honed by example, by goading, by competitive training. Then I came across a 2003 study conducted by British researcher Janet Treasure and her team at the eating disorders unit of South London's Maudsley Hospital, and my assumptions about perfectionism, eating disorders, and my own personality changed radically.

Treasure's team wanted to know whether certain early childhood traits might foreshadow anorexia and bulimia, so they devised a questionnaire to be given to patients from the unit and to a comparison sample of women who had no history of eating disorders. Most of the subjects were in their late twenties. None had any other psychiatric disorder—schizophrenia or bipolar disorder, for example—that would complicate matters. None was told the purpose of the study, nor did the questionnaire address food or body-related obsessions. Instead, the women were asked to remember habits they'd had as children that had no connection to food:

- To test for *perfectionism* the researchers asked questions like "Did you spend a long time doing and redoing your hair every morning to make sure it was straight without bumps?" They asked about each woman's childhood standards for schoolwork; the care she took of her room or pets; and other hobbies, part-time jobs, or activities. Did she have trouble in school because, no matter how many times she revised, her papers never seemed to her "good enough" to turn in? Did her friends wonder why she worked so hard?

- To gauge *inflexibility*, each woman was asked about major changes that had occurred in her childhood and how she'd responded to them. "Were you the sort of child who liked to keep a diary or written timetable? Did you need to know intricate details about an event ahead of time?" The questioners tried to determine how well each person had adapted when moving, changing schools, or shifting class schedules. Did she get upset when things did not go according to her carefully laid out plans?

- To test for attitudes toward *rules* and *discipline*, the women were asked: "Were you the kind of person who felt she always had to follow the rules? How far did you bend or break limits that were set by your parents or teachers?" Compliance and conformity were under scrutiny here, as well as attitudes about right, wrong, and rebellion.

- To test for *doubt* and *cautiousness*, the women were asked about self-doubt. "Were you frightened to make a mistake as a child?" The answer would not necessarily reflect parental pressure. Rather, the researchers were trying to get at obsessive doubts that welled up from within. They were also looking for doubt's twin: compulsive caution. "Would you rather stay home alone than risk playing an unfamiliar game with your friends?"

- Finally, the *drive for order and symmetry* was tested as a physical, even aesthetic expression of the drive for rules. "While trying to get your room tidy and organized, were you particularly concerned about making sure that everything was 'just so' and in its proper place?" Had the women felt compelled to straighten crooked pictures, line up their books, balance the light and dark clothes in their closets? Did they get upset if someone inadvertently moved their things?

But of course, I thought after reading through the categories. These habits and ways of thinking seemed so normal to me that I couldn't imagine there would be a discrepancy between the responses of the two groups. The first broad finding of this study to leap at me, then, was not the frequency of these traits among the eating disordered but their nearly total *absence* among the healthy subjects. Except for a handful who had overvalued rules and order as kids, the women who had never had eating disorders registered zero childhood perfectionism, zero inflexibility, zero doubt and cautiousness. By contrast, 60 percent of the eating disordered had been perfectionistic, rigid, and rule bound as children. A full half had qualified as inflexible, and more than one fourth had been driven by doubt, caution, and the need for symmetry.

Now, all the subjects in this study were high achievers. The healthy group consisted of students and staff recruited from two London universities, and they scored about the same as the eating disordered patients in academic performance. Yet not one of the healthy subjects remembered agonizing over grades as a child, convincing herself she wasn't good enough, or filling with rage if her friends decided to change the rules of a game. This, frankly, astonished me. Such reactions had been so typical of me as a child that I'd assumed they were true of anyone who did well in school—or, later, of anyone who succeeded professionally.

Suddenly I realized that, throughout my life, I'd generalized wildly from my particular experience, just as Caroline Knapp had in *Appetites*. Sure, I knew some people were slackers; some were party girls; and some had no particular ambitions beyond leading a quiet, comfortable life. But I had assumed that anyone who "achieved" did so with the help of an internal tyrant who established rigid standards, rules, routines, timetables, codes, and expectations. My father did. My mother did. I figured my cohorts at Yale all did, too, even if they hid it so well you couldn't tell from the outside. It never occurred to me that among other high achievers, compulsive perfectionists were the exception rather than the rule. Nor did it occur to me that my tendency to ascribe my standards to others was, in itself, a signal characteristic.

In fact, the traits highlighted in Treasure's study typify one particular personality type: obsessive-compulsive personality, or OCP. The first time I heard this term I confused it with obsessive-compulsive disorder (OCD), which is also common to some two thirds of anorexics and a third of bulimics. But although closely related, OCD and OCP belong to distinctly different categories. OCD is a type of anxiety disorder that causes uncontrollable tics and ritualistic thinking, as well as acute discomfort and shame. People with OCD might obsessively count backward, rock their bodies, or compulsively clean one spot over and over again. I do not have OCD, nor do most of my relatives. OCP, on the other hand, is undeniably my personality type, and it runs through at least three generations of my family. People with extremely obsessive-compulsive personalities not only are cautious, rigidly focused, stubborn, and perfectionistic but also tend to be quite certain that their way of acting is right and those who oppose them are wrong. They are terrified of making a mistake.

If you have an obsessive-compulsive personality you might, as I did, schedule your premarital blood tests so conscientiously early that by the time your wedding day arrives the results are no longer valid. You likely say "please," "thank you," and "excuse me" even when you're being wronged. You might work on your year-end report for weeks without progressing past the first section or spend so many weekends at the office that you miss every single one of your son's soccer games. Perhaps you boil to a rage if your mother puts even a dollop of cream in your nondairy soup. Or you so restrict your focus during a job interview that, afterward, all you can recall about your interviewer's appearance is the cherry-red necklace she was wearing. It had never occurred to me that these tendencies might relate to my eating disorder.

Janet Treasure's group did expect to see a connection, but what they did not expect was the staggering ratio that appeared when they analyzed their results: each additional childhood OCP trait multiplied the risk for anorexia nervosa by a factor of nearly seven. That meant that if you possessed all five of the traits they measured, you would be *thirty-five times* more likely to have an eating disorder than someone who happily wore mismatched socks. I more than possessed all five traits. As a child I prided myself on never returning a library book late, never missing a day of school, always having the correct change, never playing a game I couldn't win. If Treasure's findings were right, my instincts had set me up. I was made for an eating disorder.

In one of my earliest memories I am locked in battle with my mother as she tries to dress me for a costume party. She wants me to wear my winged angel outfit. I insist instead on my smocked green-and-white-checked party dress. My logic seems to me both unshakable and impeccable. The rule for parties is party dresses. Of this I am absolutely positive. I am also five years old.

That showdown represented my first Pyrrhic victory. My mother fought a good fight but could not prevail against my stubborn will. I wore my party dress. The discovery that everyone else was outfitted as a nurse or pirate or ballerina first stymied, then mortified me. The whole point of following rules was not to be wrong, not to stand out; and yet I could feel everyone staring at me, laughing (whether or not they actually were). My triumph shrank to a stone of shame that I remember viscerally to this day.

Ella Oldman, who passed through anorexia twice, first as a preteen and later in college, told me about a similar incident from her childhood. "When I was in third grade," she recalled, "I was very compulsive and always had to get the best grades. I was known as the smart kid, and I liked that. We were given honor words every week for an extra credit star with our spelling test. I'd gotten every one that year and needed one more to win the prize."

Ella's mother quizzed her the night before the test. One of the words was *scissors*. Ella spelled it correctly, but her mother didn't think so. Without bothering to consult a dictionary she said, "*Scissors* doesn't have a *c* in it."

Ella trusted her mother. "I thought I'd copied it down wrong. So on the test I spelled it incorrectly." After losing that prize she never looked up to her mother again. In her mid-thirties, she told the story as evidence that she and her mother had little in common. What seemed more obvious in the telling, however, was the ruthlessness of her perfectionism. Ella today is a tall, whip-thin woman with penetrating black eyes, abundant energy, and forceful opinions. I could tell the loss of that gold star still shamed her, much as my memory of wearing the wrong outfit to the party did me. While my memory was scored with self-contempt, however, hers was juiced with vindication. The mistake had not been hers.

Being right is vitally important to people with OCP traits. This does not always make us the most popular members of the team, but the laws of perfection rule us and we can be zealous in their defense. With an active eating disorder, these laws define perfection as thinness, creating pressure to eat less than anyone else and exercise more. At work, we may feel compelled to prove to our bosses that we can follow orders better than anyone else. We may marry someone who will put us in charge (or allow us the illusion of being in charge), or we may find no one perfect enough to suit us and so never marry. If we have children, we probably hope they won't make a mess, but we'll feel it's our fault when they do. Our instinct is to allow no exceptions, permit no one to dissuade or derail us. Of course, the greatest obstacle to perfection is our own inescapably human fallibility. The more we try to prove our infallibility, the more we are bound to fail.

Stress tends to heighten the perfectionist's appetite for order.

That is likely why so many women who are vulnerable to eating disorders develop them in prep school and college. "I knew from a girl who'd gone to Interlochen that bulimia was rampant in the dorms," Marya Hornbacher wrote of her elite private high school. "Bathrooms rarely worked because the pipes were perpetually clogged with vomit." Another young woman I met recently recalled her all-girl boarding school in England: "Out of sixty girls in the house, there were at least five anorexic girls and I don't know how many other bulimic girls. In my class of one hundred twenty, three were thin enough to be hospitalized over the course of two years." Both these schools were extremely prestigious, their student bodies intensely competitive. Rates of eating disorders on these campuses were roughly five times the national average.

But the prevalence of eating disorders at high-pressure schools is now common knowledge. What's less widely recognized is the frequency of relapse later in life during stressful events such as career transitions and relationship breakups. The resurgence of Candace Lunt's anorexia in midlife coincided with both. Restricting her diet to one thousand calories a day gave her an illusion of control as she left her husband and risked moving three thousand miles to take a challenging new job. Six years later, though, reflecting on it with me one evening after dinner at her apartment in Manhattan, she could point to the moment when she realized that perfectionism, far from being the answer to her problems, was actually her biggest handicap.

She recalled the wait in her office at *Forbes* for her boss to arrive for her first performance review. Just one month earlier she'd separated from her husband in San Francisco and brought six-year-old Ruby to an apartment in midtown New York that Candace could barely afford. Now her ex-husband was demanding she pay *him* alimony. *Luck is opportunity met with preparedness,* her screen saver blinked. This was one of the sayings that had persuaded her to convert to Judaism before leaving San Francisco. The principle of accountability, as she understood it from her readings of the Jewish texts, had brought her a profound sense of relief and hope. After forty years, she finally understood that she was not responsible for the choices other people made. She was, however, *accountable* for her own choices and responses to the people around her. Her religious conversion had emboldened her to risk this career advance, stop using excuses to hold herself back, and reach unapologetically for a change—becoming a senior editor at a national publication—that she was absolutely certain she wanted.

Taking such risks was alien to her nature, however, and she could feel herself wrestling this nature every inch of the way. Her move to New York had been precipitated by the loss of a major promotion at the *San Francisco Chronicle*—a promotion her bosses there had assured her was hers for the taking. "So I was beating myself up for having allowed them to walk all over me," she told me, "and then in the process trying to nail all these changes. I wouldn't let myself eat until I'd proved I could pull this off. The dropped pounds were my reward, visible proof of progress. It was like going for the straight A average while losing thirty pounds my junior year in high school. It was all about cleaning up my act, sharpening my performance, and buying a new start."

I started to object. No one's performance is *really* at its sharpest during a crash diet. But Candace signaled me to hold on.

Her new job at *Forbes*, she said, put her in charge of a department of eight. She had prepared herself with lists, flowcharts, sets of clear rules and expectations. She arrived early, left late, and didn't eat lunch. She kept her door shut so she could concentrate and asked that her staff schedule all meetings in advance. She color coded her files; alphabetized her lists; and set up a numerical system for tracking past, present, and potential assignments. She was haunted by memories of her apartment in San Francisco before she left her marriage: dust balls, dying aspidistras, old phone messages, and to-do lists filled with jobs that had gone undone. "There were corners of such mess and neglect. It wasn't happy. It wasn't cohesive." She was determined that her new office and home would be clean, orderly, and controlled. But the result of her efforts was that she became increasingly invisible. "I was hiding. I knew it. I hadn't broken through that wall."

This sounded like Marya Hornbacher's barrier, that mirror-thin wall that concealed the real person behind the glass.

"Finally my boss came in and sat me down. He was a tough, grizzled newsman, and when he put you on the hot seat you knew it. He glared at me for what felt like an hour. Then he said, 'As a manager here you define yourself by the way you extend yourself. You have to create your own management style—your own legacy in your own time. If you don't do that, you drown very quickly and become a nobody.' He stopped. I knew what was coming, but nothing can prepare you. He said, 'I don't think I'm getting my money's worth. I hired you because I thought you were going to be a brilliant manager, and you're not.' "

Candace wanted to defend herself. She was responsible, vigilant, attentive to detail, scrupulously honest, and the hardest worker on staff. Competent to the point of compulsiveness, she had a stellar résumé and an excellent record. No one had ever spoken to her like this before. But that was precisely why she could not bring herself to speak now. When her marriage broke up, her husband had begged her not to leave—even as he cleaned out their bank account. Her previous employers had unfailingly praised her, while lying about her being slated for promotion. The teachers who put her on the honor roll never acknowledged her visible emaciation. Nor did her parents. Now, on this April evening in New York when she was forty-four years old, Candace was as stunned by her boss's unbridled honesty as she was panicked by his attack. This was not like getting an A- instead of A+. Across the board and with potentially devastating consequences, she had failed by doing everything in her power to prove the perfectionist was in control.

"I just sat there," Candace remembered, "waiting for the final blow."

Instead, her boss said, "I know you *want* to be a creative manager."

Recalling her shock in the moment, Candace covered her mouth, but then let her hand drop as she laughed out loud. "He was going to give me another chance!"

She pushed back in her wooden rocking chair and glanced with a look of wonder at the touchstone objects that filled her living room now—seedpods, feathers, a sculptural twist of tree bark, an inlaid mandolin, and artwork by Ruby and friends. Candace and Ruby live in a small two-bedroom apartment in lower Manhattan. Everything is orderly but not impeccably so. In the year since we'd first reconnected in New Mexico, Candace had let her hair go gray. It hung straight as raw silk to her shoulders, softening her face. Her body, too, seemed softer, more settled. She was fifty and not fighting it. That evening the whole apartment held the aroma of curried salmon, an improvised recipe Candace had prepared for our dinner with Ruby, who was now doing her homework down the hall. Succeeding under her new boss, Candace said, had meant changing her whole outlook, dropping the pretense of controlled perfection, developing a level of flexibility that was alien to both her nature and the way she'd been raised. She had to learn to think creatively, even to welcome change. Most important of all, she had to come out of hiding.

Candace created what she called "artificial conditions," but which, in reality, were the undoing of conditions that came naturally only to her. She had to leave her phone and e-mail, emerge from her office, and meet with her staff in person; keep her door open and encourage people to come to her with problems; learn to listen when they told her why they'd missed a deadline; address their problems honestly and directly; confront when necessary to keep her staff thinking; figure out and express what she honestly believed was best for the larger enterprise—the magazine that carried all their names on the masthead. She had to remind herself over and over that failure is not insurmountable; sometimes it's absolutely necessary. Often it leads to change for the better.

Candace couldn't tell me exactly when she began to regain the twenty pounds she'd lost in transition. By the time she noticed she was back to normal, she was immersed in her job and getting Ruby settled in school. She no longer needed to deny herself in order to prove she was in control. The upshot of this reversal still surprised her, even as we talked about it. "I'm sure a lot of people with my personality go through life choosing careers where they won't have to deal with confrontation and uncertainty, but I had chosen one that put all this stuff on the table. I had some big, gaping holes that had to be reconciled. My job forced me not only to resolve them but to excel at resolving them."

She rocked back in her chair and sighed. "It's like teaching expressiveness and trust. To teach it, I first had to learn it myself."

If you are a perfectionist, your instinct is to perform flawlessly or else, in your mind, you're a failure. This is why criticism feels so threatening. It's also why perfectionists tend to excel when standards are clear and crisp, as in school or sports or jobs like accounting, engineering, or science. When standards shift or call for flexibility, perfectionists tend to falter. As the risk for error rises, so does the perfectionist's anxiety level. Candace knew she was taking a chance when she made her career move, since her natural instinct when anxious was to tighten her grip. To succeed as an editor she had to learn to do precisely the opposite: relax. Her terror of criticism made this almost impossible. Yet, paradoxically, she needed that criticism in order to change. As devastating as her boss's judgment seemed at the time, it was a gift of honest generosity and truth.

What Candace experienced on the job—the simultaneous needs to achieve absolute control and to break free of that control—mirrors the internal contradictions of perfectionism. The emotional promise of perfection is security: no one will criticize you, try to change you, or touch you if you have your universe in order. But because perfection is impossible, frustration is inevitable and at times unbearable. One feels simultaneously like the horse pulling forward and the rider pulling back on the reins. While a wise boss can release the reins in a work situation, internally each of us must act as our own psychological boss. Eating disorders actually serve this internal boss by reducing the need for perfection to a manageable scale: the body. But for perfectionists who have renounced eating disorders, the brain must rely on substitute methods. One is nail biting.

When I called my old classmate Yvonne Anderson to ask how she treated her hands, there was a long pause. Over the phone I couldn't tell if she was thinking or annoyed. Finally she burst out in embarrassed laughter. "You have *got* to be kidding!" She'd tried everything, she said, from chewing gum to worry beads, but in fifty years she'd found nothing that would rid her of the habit. Nail biting was another of those secret, shameful compulsions, like starving and purging, that Yvonne had never even talked about. Curiously, what most bothers her about these habits is the very thing that makes them habitual: the sensation of zoning out. The preoccupation with her hands acts "like a wall," she observed, like Candace echoing Hornbacher, "to keep me from fully experiencing life, just as fasting used to."

I knew what she meant. The effect is like drifting in space. While ostensibly reading, you absorb nothing from the page. If standing in a group of people, you stop hearing what they say. If arguing with your husband, you mentally absent yourself from the fight. All the anxiety of the situation pours into your fingers—and out of your head and heart. Just when you most want or need to pay attention, you effectively disappear.

This bizarre, disfiguring habit, paradoxically, is rooted in grooming behavior. The primitive urge to bite, tear, fiddle with our nails begins with the need to fix or perfect ourselves. It is reinforced, in humans as in our primate relatives, by chemistry. Most nail biters probably don't realize that this "nervous habit" has a distinct physiological effect on the brain, but of course that effect is the very reason we tug at our nails (and perhaps hair, too) when anxious. Nail biting, like bingeing, purging, and fasting, alters the activity of the neurotransmitter serotonin in the brain. For some people this can have the effect of releasing tension.

Normally, serotonin helps to modulate mood, anxiety, appetite, and sexuality. The chemical becomes most active in the face of danger, when it triggers the fight-or-flight instinct. It heightens fear, short-circuits hunger and libido, and narrows one's focus to the imminent threat. But researchers have found that people with histories of anorexia and, to a lesser extent, bulimia have high serotonin levels even when no physical threat is present. These levels shape not just their anxiety levels but their personality. "Typically well organized, driven, and somewhat compulsive," Peter Kramer writes in *Listening to Prozac*, "they are extremely obedient and may overachieve in school, even in the face of disrupted home lives. They are good at following through on tasks, tend to sleep too much rather than too little, are rarely impulsive or domineering, and, indeed, tend to be timid and risk-averse. They do better in the face of routine and worse in the face of novelty. And they are prone to depression."

Fasting reduces serotonin activity. With prolonged dieting or severe weight loss, however, the levels may drop too low, intensifying depression and creating a desperate sense of impulsiveness. A binge will raise serotonin activity, but usually too fast and too high, now prompting a purge. As University of Pittsburgh professor Walter Kaye explained it to me, the eating disordered are forever chasing a sensation of comfort they never can quite catch. This chase typically is occurring, Kaye believes, long before an eating disorder begins, and it continues long after recovery. Hence the persistence of substitute habits like nail biting.

In 2004 National Institute of Mental Health (NIMH) researchers identified a rare gene mutation shared by people with anorexia nervosa, OCD, and obsessive-compulsive personality disorder, the most rigid extreme of OCP. This mutation, which creates an imbalance in serotonin activity, may help to explain why eating disorders, perfectionism, and depression so frequently overlap. About half of all women with anorexia nervosa and at least one fourth of bulimics will suffer from major depression at some point in their lives, and some, like the writer Virginia Woolf, become anorexic *only* when depressed. What's interesting about Woolf's anorexia, though, is that it was not simply a loss of appetite or an inability to eat but a true fat fixation—a fixation that ran in her family. According to her biographer, Mitchell Leaska, "The worst problem during the first week was food. She was convinced that she was fat and ugly, that there was something disgusting about food and eating. When the nurses came near her with meals she grew violent. They must leave her alone! Had Leonard [her husband] not taken endless hours coaxing one spoonful of food at a time, at all three meals each day, she would probably have died of starvation just as her cousin James Kenneth Stephen had twenty-one years earlier at St. Andrew's Hospital."

If Virginia Woolf and her cousin lived today they would likely be treated with Prozac, Celexa, or another of the drugs collectively known as selective serotonin reuptake inhibitors (SSRIs). Although these antidepressants appear to have little effect on severely underweight anorexics, they are frequently prescribed to combat depression, obsessive-compulsive behavior, and bulimia following weight recovery. For several of the men and women I interviewed, SSRIs have become a normal and necessary part of their daily regimen.

A dog barked when I rang the bell of the Andersons' Seattle home. Yvonne had to straddle Rex, her golden retriever, to hold him back as she opened the door. This Ph.D. in comparative religion and mother of two teenagers wore jean overalls, a magenta T-shirt, flip-flops with huge dahlias blooming between her toes, and her long, prematurely white hair pulled high into a ponytail. It was an unseasonably warm September afternoon, and she was just back from a "walking meditation." As she gave me a hug I registered, still, the angular spareness of her body, but her mood was irrepressible.

We settled to talk in her favorite room, a library that held two solid walls of books. "We just sit here after dinner, and our eyes feast," Yvonne said.

I followed her gaze, tracing a course of literary history from Cervantes to Dave Eggers, with stops in every major religion and political movement along the way. Faith and activism had become the dominant themes in Yvonne's life. My question was how the silent, withdrawn anorexic I'd known in school had come to make this transition.

"It was always there, just . . ." She paused for a moment, then detoured to the subject of her morning's meditation. "I was drawn to the sun. So I sat down and looked into these chimes. It felt like sunbathing when I was growing up. How peaceful. We used to waste so much time sunbathing, but I didn't feel like I was wasting time. Back then it was so easy, so natural just to be. I think my transition, as you put it, has been my whole life, trying to get back to that sense of peace." Alas, in the aftermath of war, peace becomes relative, at best. This is as true for veterans of anorexia and bulimia as it is for veterans of Vietnam or Iraq.

Yvonne offered me a diet Snapple. It was understood, even now, that neither of us would consider drinking a *non* diet drink. Then we compared our gnawed fingernails and cuticles. Yvonne shook her head, recalling our phone conversation about anorexia and nail biting. "I can put on a good show. It helps remind me what I'm aiming for, but none of it comes easy."

I knew. Back when we were in school, Yvonne wore her despair like a uniform. With her long cayenne-red hair and posture trained by years of ballet, she cut a striking figure as she strode across campus, but she rarely spoke to a soul. I monitored her from afar, the same way I did Candy Lunt and Kim Olensky, noting the way she buried her body in overalls, the bite-size portions she arranged on her plate, the tight stretch of her skin over bone. With her sunken eyes and cheeks Yvonne in her teens had looked sixty.

"I did my senior thesis in college on poets' responses to death, which pretty much sums up my outlook on life my entire adolescence. I didn't expect to live past my twenties, and frankly I didn't want to."

Depression runs deep in Yvonne's family. Even before she began to sense it in herself as a teenager, she could feel her father's suffering. Her dad was her role model, an inspiring social organizer, and community leader. But he also had a melancholy side, often retreating into solitude. When Yvonne wanted to talk to him, she had to make an appointment. His first wife had been killed in a car accident—when he was driving—and neither Yvonne's mother nor his two daughters ever fully penetrated his guilt and grief.

Cause or effect? With depression, as with eating disorders, the question of what comes first creates a loop of inquiry. But the fact is, not everyone who survives a car crash, callous parents, childhood abuse, or other trauma necessarily suffers chronic depression. A provocative World Health Organization survey of fourteen nations conducted in 2004 found that Nigerians—with an average annual income of $300, epidemic numbers of HIV-positive people and cases of AIDS, and a life expectancy of just forty-five years—have a lower rate of depression than residents of any Western or Asian country, while America, with all its affluence and medical advances, has the highest rate, more than eleven times higher than Nigeria's. Possible explanations for such difference range from genetics to diet to sociology, but the cruel truth is that all people are not equally resilient to the everyday stresses of life, let alone to catastrophic loss. Even within the ranks of the depressed, as Andrew Solomon writes in *The Noonday Demon,* "Willfulness and pride may allow one person to get through a depression that would fell another whose personality is more gentle and acquiescent. Depression interacts with personality."

Willfulness and pride being hallmarks of their personality, perfectionists do tend to "get through" depression. Yvonne's father, for example, lived into his eighties and never sought treatment for his black moods. But stoicism is no ticket to health or happiness. Yvonne and her sister, Wanda, both grew up acutely aware of the darkness their father carried inside him, especially after they began to recognize that same darkness within themselves.

Wanda, now a lawyer, was always more outgoing than Yvonne. She never had anorexia or bulimia, but she did obsess about her health. She shopped only at organic food stores; swallowed supplements by the fistful; ate food only in its rawest form; and abstained from animal fat, refined sugar, white flour, saturated oils. She became a lacto-ovo vegetarian, then a vegan. As the scope of her diet shrank, she stopped eating out with friends. She argued with her husband and children over what she would and would not eat and "the garbage they put in their mouths." When not shopping for the perfect lettuce, she played tennis up to four hours a day; visited the doctor, sometimes four times a week; and monitored her medical records the same way Yvonne used to monitor her weight. None of Wanda's ultra-healthy practices, however, stopped her from worrying. In her late forties she became convinced she was losing her memory, experiencing early-onset Alzheimer's. She expanded her rounds of doctors, traveling across country to specialists. They told her she had a condition called orthorexia, a "fixation on righteous eating" that turns health food into an unhealthy obsession. They also told her that, in fact, she *had* suffered memory loss, but not because of Alzheimer's. What made Wanda forgetful was her terror of forgetting.

Yvonne laughed as she described her sister's intensity, but it was a laugh of empathy. Yvonne relies on her students, family, doctor, and minister to help her keep her own health in check, but like her sister she is constantly afraid of doing something wrong. "I can never be good enough," she told me—the perfectionist's refrain.

To illustrate the point, Yvonne told me about an evening a few years earlier that should have made her feel she'd reached a pinnacle in her life. She was moving with her family from the town where they had lived for over five years, and the students and faculty of her college threw her a farewell party. Dozens turned out to thank Yvonne and bid her good-bye, and the party went on for hours. Thoughts of her mistakes hounded her all evening. "It was too much to bear," she told me. "After I left I was shaking and crying so hard I had to stop the car on the way home." The outpouring of love had triggered intense feelings of guilt—the conviction that she did not deserve this love. She couldn't stop replaying the evening, how she had failed to talk to one person or should have hugged another. How she'd said the wrong thing in her remarks, failed to thank the right people, forgotten to get back to that woman who was waiting so patiently. . . . Yvonne knows this sense of failure is as irrational as her sister's obsession with memory loss. She also realizes that their thought patterns are related. "It's a genetic curse," Yvonne said.

I studied my friend's dahlia flip-flops, considered the photographs of her beaming face during a recent family trip to Kenya, the volumes around us that she treasured. "No one would ever guess."

"Maybe. But get this: when I first started on antidepressants, I went to a psychopharmacologist to make sure we found the right medication, dosage, minimal side effects, all that? He started me on Celexa. It turned out Wanda was already taking exactly the same drug."

Identifying just the right type and dosage of medication,

however, is an ongoing process. Yvonne's primary complaint about antidepressants is their tendency to suppress libido. "It surprises me even now, but in all these years of struggling with my weight and mood, one gift for me has been my body's enjoyment of giving and receiving pleasure." Unwilling to surrender that pleasure, she at first tried to work around the medication by "taking vacations," skipping her pills Friday through Sunday in order to enjoy weekends with her husband. "But then Monday comes, and I think, this is okay. And I don't take them Monday or Tuesday, and by Wednesday, I can feel the darkness descending. And then it's so hard to get back to normal." More recently she's been trying the newer SSRIs in hopes of reducing this side effect. "The latest is Effexor. We'll see."

While medication helps to calm her moods, Yvonne stressed, it does not change her habits of thought. So she has developed her own brand of behavior modification to counter her instinctive self-loathing. She refuses to read fashion magazines. She won't allow herself to diet, spends minimal time in front of the mirror, and doesn't own a scale. "I will not weigh myself, which is also frankly anorexic, but if I knew how much I weighed, it would be too easy for me to say I want to weigh less. This way I don't think about the number." She guesses her weight to be about 140 but depends on the fit of her clothes to tell her when she needs to exercise a little more or less. Tennis she plays because she loves it and because it's a social sport. She also meditates and does yoga to calm her mind.

All these strategies, however, are secondary to faith in what Yvonne calls "the daily struggle to stay in touch with the joy of life." Though she recalls having a strong belief in God during childhood, her faith receded when she was anorexic. After college, when she hit her turning point and decided she had to come back to life, she chose sacred music over psychotherapy. Though she'd never been treated for her own eating disorder, she led a music therapy program for anorexic hospital patients. She studied Sufi and Hassidic traditions, and entered divinity school. After earning her doctorate, Yvonne served as a chaplain for juveniles in detention before returning to academia as a professor of theology.

"My faith saved my life," she told me. She was quick to add, however, that not even faith had "cured" her. "I still don't trust my own signals."

By signals, Yvonne meant those pesky traits that are ruled by temperament—her anxiety about never being good enough, her need for approval, her reluctance to risk failure, her tendency to work herself into the ground. Antidepressants help physiologically. Church provides the emotional safety nets of prayer, community, and spiritual counsel. But most important, she told me, "Redemption comes in channeling that need to be most perfect into compassion and acceptance—for others as well as myself."

"Do you ever regret those anorexic years?"

The phone rang. She stared at it, letting the machine pick up. "I won't allow myself to go there. If I regret too much, I won't live in the moment. I try instead to turn regret into redemption. The old Carl Jung phrase 'There's no coming to consciousness without pain.' Coming to consciousness, listening to who you are and living out of that place—that, for me, is what it's all about."

Yvonne's return to health depended as much on character as on chemistry, and by character I mean not toughness or moral fiber but the aspects of personality that one shapes by choice. Seeking effective treatment is an act of character, as is the exploration of faith, the commitment to marriage and parenthood, and active participation in a congregation. The will to change is character's fuel, full consciousness its reward.

According to Washington University psychiatrist Robert Cloninger, who has been studying the biology of personality for more than twenty years, character is the real stuff of recovery because it consists of the traits we *can* change—unlike temperament,* which is largely innate and permanent. If one thinks of temperament as the genetic wiring of personality, then character consists of the circuit boards that route, suppress, or maximize the currents flowing through that wiring. The three traits that comprise character—self-directedness, self-transcendence, and cooperativeness—are shaped less by genetics than by experience (how we are raised by our parents, for example, or trained by our culture) and free will (how we choose to interpret and react to experience).

Directly or indirectly, these traits are the focus of every social organization the world over, from tribes and clans to churches, corporations, and twelve-step programs. All operate by marshaling individuals to work together effectively for a greater purpose. Ideally, this focus benefits the individual by helping her see how she fits into the larger world, reassuring her that she's not alone, and reinforcing her strengths while helping her to overcome her weaknesses. Sometimes, however, the manipulation of character creates an illusion of perfection that instead thwarts the individual. Cults that condition members to subvert themselves for the benefit of a charismatic leader are perhaps the most extreme example, but plenty of others exist within the social mainstream. A sorority, for instance, may pressure each pledge to conform to a signature look and body size, no matter how radically this requires her to distort her natural style and physique. Or die-hard family tradition may require that every child in the clan become a doctor—even the one who has been turning out exquisite drawings and failing

---

* The four inborn traits that comprise temperament in Cloninger's model are:

1. *Novelty seeking*, which determines our appetite for new experiences and excitement (typically low in perfectionists)

2. *Harm avoidance*, which controls our capacity for risk taking (high in perfectionists)

3. *Reward dependence*, which shapes our need to please others (usually moderate to low in perfectionists)

4. *Persistence*, which determines our ability to work toward long-term goals (high in perfectionists)

math and science since she was six. Character can be either cultivated or crushed by others, be they well-meaning parents or domineering friends. Ultimately, individual health demands that we recognize these traits as personal assets and claim responsibility for nurturing them ourselves.

In his book *Feeling Good: The Science of Well-Being*, Cloninger writes that the first trait of character, *self-directedness*, can be measured by the degree of meaning and purpose we feel in our lives. This sense of direction has less to do with *what*, specifically, we want than with *why* we want it. Two young women apply to graduate school: The one who lacks self-direction applies because her best friend is going, while her self-directed classmate loves marine biology so much that she can hardly wait to study the molecular workings of tide pools. Highly self-directed people like Yvonne Anderson and Candace Lunt are realistic about their abilities, effective in their choices, and persistent in solving their own problems. Instead of blaming others, they hold themselves accountable and take pride in their reliability. Self-directedness, however, is not the same as self-sufficiency. Quite the contrary, being self-directed allows us to work, play, and be intimate with others without fearing that we will lose ourselves in the process. For this reason, *cooperativeness*, the character trait that makes us feel part of society, actually benefits from self-directedness.

Highly cooperative people find that their personal passions and talents flourish within group situations. That grad student in marine biology is more likely to make a stunning discovery about plankton when working with a team than she is in isolation. Through cooperation she's also more likely to develop her capacity for empathy, tolerance, and compassion for others while gaining a broader perspective on herself. Connecting in this way was a central challenge for Candace in her managerial position and for Yvonne with her students. Like most people with a history of anorexia, both women instinctively tended to be loners, but the confidence and support they have gained by opening themselves to others has relieved the pressure of perfectionism and soothed their innate anxiety.

In its largest sense, this process of opening defines *self-transcendence*. This third character trait allows us to feel part of the greater universe. Self-transcendence gives us faith. It alleviates fear. According to Cloninger, it is a measure of "the depths of self-aware consciousness, such as awareness of what it means to see the colors of a rainbow or the beauty of a painting. . . . Individuals high in self-transcendence recognize the beauty and meaning in sensory experiences intuitively." By cultivating self-transcendence through prayer, meditation, art, music, and their respective religious studies, Yvonne and Candace both found sources of meaning beyond material possessions and appearances. They also tapped into sources of resilience and hope.

The struggle between who we are and who we want to be is what motivates most human beings to grow. The danger for perfectionists with a history of eating disorders is that they will try to change themselves by killing themselves—physically, emotionally, or spiritually. Instead of protesting fashion's ludicrous insistence that grown women wear size 4, they will shrink themselves to size 0. Instead of challenging a belligerent husband, they will silence themselves. Instead of confronting a boss who overworks them, they will sacrifice their personal life to prove that they can take any amount of punishment. Unfortunately, what perfectionists strive to prove is impossible. No one is perfect, and everyone has limits. What kills us will not make us stronger or prettier or more lovable. A sense of purpose, connection, and perspective, however, can and will.

When I graduated from college I made a conscious decision to test my preconceptions about who I had to be and what I had to do in life. In effect, though I didn't realize it at the time, I was attempting to rehabilitate my character after its long, withering anorexic siege. Determined to be self-reliant, to live on my own in New York City and support myself financially, I had to admit that a degree in painting and a typing speed of five words per minute (most of which contained typos) did not make me a strong candidate for the business world. But I discovered that I could wait tables. The money was good enough, and waitressing allowed me time to do what I most wanted to do, which was to paint and write. The work also taught me more than my Ivy League education ever had about cooperativeness. A waitress gets no tips if she can't work smoothly with her cook, busboy, bartender, and fellow waitstaff. If she's flexible enough to fill in for someone else, then that person might help her out on a night when she can't work. These were lessons that I might have learned years earlier had I gone in for team sports, belonged to more youth groups, or grown up in a less individualistic culture or generation. (Current studies show that girls who play on teams are less likely to develop eating disorders than girls who engage in solo sports like track or swimming, and this element of cooperativeness may be one reason why.) But like most girls of my generation, I had little experience in teams, and like most perfectionists, I tended to join only clubs that I could single-handedly control. The combined effort it took to run a restaurant was a revelation to me.

Then I heard that United was hiring flight attendants. The higher salary and free travel appealed to me, and I enjoyed the bemused looks I got from Yale classmates when they learned I'd become a "stew."

Flying forced me to reconsider the stress I placed on perfection. Once, when I was in the rear jump seat of a chartered stretch DC-8 coming into Pensacola, we hit the tarmac so violently my shoulder harnesses flew off—hardly a flawless landing. But the runway in Pensacola then was dangerously short for long planes like ours, which is why they didn't ordinarily land there. As the pilot later explained, touching down smoothly might well have landed us in the ocean at the end of the runway. He had to choose between protecting our nerves and protecting our lives. Then there was the packed DC-10 trip out of

JFK when a snafu in the galley delayed the meal service for nearly a full hour. The trays were still in front of the passengers as we taxied up to the jetway at O'Hare, and some nasty "onion letters" were doubtless sent to United that day, but no one was injured, no one fired. In the grand scheme of things, it was a survivable screwup.

Such lessons did not affect my preference for straight lines, orderly closets, or games I know I can win. They did shake up my rigidity, however, and force me to recognize that imperfection does not have to be a terminal offense. Error sometimes supplies the surprise that makes life interesting. Sometimes it opens up new opportunities. There's a good reason why we rarely remember, much less tell stories about, the perfect landings.

4

WANTING FOR NOTHING

Avoidance

Health is not associated with *denial* of anything.
—D. W. Winnicott

ONE WARM SPRING DAY near the end of my junior year in college—after I'd decided to resume normal life but before I'd made much tangible progress—I joined two seniors I admired as they picnicked on Science Hill. Lia was an economics major. She had straight, cropped, no-nonsense brown hair and an aquiline nose. Her penetrating blue eyes had mesmerized more than a few of my male classmates. Jen was graduating with a combined degree in political science and African studies. A redhead with a boy's haircut, she was as bony as I was but easy in her body. She attacked her lunch of take-out sandwiches, chips, and soda—not Tab or Fresca but root beer—with the appetite of a wolf. Lia, by comparison, inhaled her food as if eating was as natural as breathing. We all wore jeans and T-shirts, no makeup. From a distance we must have looked like three of a kind, but while Lia and Jen stretched out on the grass, I sat with my arms wrapped around my knees, unable to uncoil.

"You want some?" Lia asked with her mouth full, holding out her package of Fritos. I shook my head, lied that I'd eaten. She took a slug of Coke. Everything about Lia was matter-of-fact, even the way she put on her horn-rimmed glasses, as something she needed to do in order to read, to learn, to think, to decide what she wanted to do next. So it took me by surprise when she admitted she wasn't sure what she was going to do after graduation. "The admissions office has offered me a job for the summer, but I feel like I ought to get out of here. My father's pushing me to take the GREs in case I decide to go to grad school, and all I really want to do is bum around Europe for a couple of months."

"Count me in!" Jen grinned. "If you'll pay back my student loans so I don't have to work in my stepfather's law firm."

As Lia chewed her tuna fish sandwich, I was calculating that one bite contained fifty calories, five grams of carbohydrates, and four grams of fat. The mayonnaise made the waxed paper glint in the bright sun. I tried to imagine not noticing the oil, not thinking about the water weight the salt from the Fritos would cause. I tried to understand how Lia could ignore what she was putting into her mouth and focus on her future. My own future beyond my last remaining year of school looked as blank as an empty plate.

Jen offered this advice: Lia should accept the job in the admissions office for the summer and take the Graduate Record Exams in August, then split for Europe in the fall, after the tourist season. "Have your cake and eat it, too."

"I never really thought about that." My voice startled us all. Lia tilted her head, not understanding. "I mean that saying. It never made sense to me."

"For it to make sense," Jen said pointedly, "you have to admit you want the cake."

I thought about Jen's remark often over the next two years as I slowly repositioned myself for life beyond graduation. All three of us that day had been engaged in a calculation of needs and means, desired gains and necessary sacrifices. These were not all-or-nothing choices. But they were choices that required us to know what we wanted.

I thought of Jen's remark again thirty years later as I listened to a fifty-year-old Chicago housewife named Lucy Romanello describe her ambivalence about wanting. "I'll punish myself," Lucy told me, "because I don't feel close to God when I feel full or I've indulged. I love sixteenth-century sacred music, for example, but if I'm disgusted with myself, I won't let myself listen."

Jen, I suspected, would have had little patience with Lucy. My reaction was more perplexed. I'd met Lucy online when she replied to the note on my Web site asking for interview volunteers. At first, as we spoke by phone and e-mailed, her story sounded familiar. Thirty years earlier, while a sophomore at NYU, she had dieted down to 85 pounds. At her college counselor's insistence she was hospitalized and attended twelve-step meetings, but she found these sessions more harmful than helpful because the group members tended to be so competitive and often described methods for purging or weight loss that Lucy proceeded to try. It was not a prescribed treatment that ultimately worked for her. Instead, she fell in love with a colleague at work, a "younger man" by two years. He had a wry sense of humor and thought she was funny. Then he saw her refrigerator, empty except for a can of Tab and a jar of mustard, and he asked if she was okay. "I was too embarrassed to keep starving," she told me. "I didn't want to lose him." Lucy married her man, now an advertising executive with J. Walter Thompson, and they chose not to have children. She worked as a bookkeeper until, at forty, she decided to get a master's degree in theology. In divinity school she earned straight A's, as she had in college, and graduated with honors. But at this point Lucy's history deviated from the usual perfectionist pattern. With her husband's support, she chose not to return to work. Other than Mondays, when she volunteered in the soup kitchen at her church, for the past nine years she had spent the bulk of her days alone. "I read," she told me. "I listen to music. In nice weather I walk around town." Except, she added, when she feels too disgusted with herself.

Superficially, Lucy reminded me of Yvonne Anderson. Both were devout Episcopalians who had excelled in divinity school and, as Lucy put it, sought "self-transcendence through a relationship with Jesus Christ." Both had recovered from anorexia in their early twenties, around the time they married, and both had been married to the same men ever since. But while Yvonne had graduated from seminary into a busy life of teaching, motherhood, marriage, and community, Lucy had chosen to retreat from society. Her life as she described it made me think not of Yvonne's abundant household but of Kim Olensky's underfurnished white condo by the beach. The difference, I suspected, had less to do with faith than it did with temperament. I decided to meet Lucy in person.

She chose a small, sedate restaurant down the block from her church in Chicago's South Loop so that she could meet me directly for lunch after serving at the soup kitchen. She was sitting ramrod straight in a quiet corner when I arrived. Her black hair shimmered with early gray, falling straight to her shoulders, not a strand out of place, her nails manicured short and naked as a nun's. Lucy's figure was slight, her makeup almost undetectable, and her large blue-gray eyes studied me intently. Though fifty, she looked ill at ease in her powder-blue sweater set and pearls, as if she were wearing her mother's clothes.

We reviewed the little I knew about her Baltimore childhood from our phone conversations. Her father was an appliance salesman who used to discipline Lucy and her younger sister with his belt buckle. Her mother was a special education teacher who often berated Lucy with the appalling comment "You're worse than my retards." When Lucy was in elementary school her parents forbade her to play with her best friend because the girl was Jewish and her mother divorced. Lucy heeded her parents' restrictions but also rebelled by drawing into herself, avoiding family gatherings and parties. Her plunge in weight was a reaction to her father's teasing about her thick waist when she came home from her freshman year at college. Her parents, however, didn't get the message. Lucy's overweight mother actually told her she looked great standing five-foot-six and weighing 89 pounds.

The waiter chose this inauspicious moment to ask for our order. I automatically chose a salad; Lucy requested a roast beef sandwich. She explained she had to eat red meat to make up for the damage done to her body during her anorexic years. "I have the bones of a seventy-five-year-old. I've lost half an inch of height and broken two bones in the last ten months." She'd begun taking calcium and working out with weights, but she feared the damage was permanent, as was her sensitivity to cold, which she also traced back to her eating disorder. During Chicago's brutal winters, she said, she often went weeks without leaving her apartment.

I, too, am cold averse (though my bones, so far, remain strong). The winter I was based in Chicago while working for United, the windchill factor brought temperatures down to thirty below, and the next year I moved to Southern California. Still, I could not imagine living as insular an existence as Lucy's, regardless the temperature outside. "What keeps you going?" I asked her.

"My faith." The reply came so fast it sounded rehearsed.

Here, I had to confess my own agnosticism. I was baptized and confirmed on the same day at a small community church when I was thirteen, and I had not attended services since. In college I studied East Asian religions, and if I had to adopt a faith it would be either Buddhism or Unitarian Universalism. However, I've never felt the pull of organized religion, never experienced the need for a church or high priest to mediate my relationship with God.

Lucy nodded. "My family's not religious either. My mother still thinks I'm some kind of freak for going to church. But I remember being a really little girl and writing prayers on slips of paper and throwing them out the window and thinking they'd fly up to heaven." As a teenager she attended church by herself. "The Episcopal church gave me the kind of unconditional love I never felt growing up."

I asked her to help me understand how she could ever be "disgusting," a word she'd used over and over during our correspondence, in the eyes of a God who loved her unconditionally.

"I love things that are beautiful. That's part of the appeal of church—the beauty of holiness. So when I eat a lot—not even bingeing, just eating more than I should—I feel disgusting to myself, and then I feel that I must be disgusting to God."

It struck me as Lucy continued that this disgust might have more to do with her parents than with God. "My parents would tell me I was such a disappointment," she said. "I could never do anything right. My parents and sister seemed happy being extroverted and superficial, while I was introverted and spiritual. If I ever dared express this aspect of my personality, I was mocked."

"Your husband's different, I take it?"

"My husband's another loner. But he made me feel really good about myself, even when I was anorexic."

Our lunch arrived. Lucy picked up her sandwich and dutifully began to eat. I asked her to tell me more about her marriage. "What happens, for instance, when you argue?"

She grinned and wiped her mouth. "I'm horrible at it. Whenever we have a fight, he goes on a rant, screaming; and even if he's wrong I usually just sit there, and then I'll start crying, and that's the end of the fight."

Since I'd done the same thing through most of my marriage, we began comparing notes. I'd kept so many of my thoughts and feelings to myself I'd effectively led a secret life. So had Lucy. Sometimes her husband would talk for hours and she wouldn't open her mouth. I told her I had trouble asking for what I really wanted, especially sexually, but I had developed other passions, for painting and writing and, more recently, photography. Lucy said her passion was church. But had the church helped her

stand up for herself? She shook her head. "I am still so introverted and so unwilling to bother anybody, and I am so—so
afraid of confrontation. When I'm around people who have
very different opinions from mine, I won't engage. I get really
tense even watching other people debate or argue."

Lucy had hated her career, which consisted mostly of clerical
and accounting tasks, but she'd hated being promoted more because it always seemed to land her in a management position.
"I couldn't even tell a woman who reported to me and who was
an hour late every morning, 'Please come to work on time.' "
Now she avoids leadership at all costs: "Even at the soup
kitchen, the person who is in charge will ask me to fill in for her
while she's on vacation, and I say no!" Lucy laughed at this, at
herself, as if apologizing.

I thought of Candace hiding in her office, dwelling on her
files to avoid confronting her staff. But she had finally—albeit
under threat of termination—chosen to learn how to engage.
Lucy seemed almost willful in her *dis*engagement.

I asked what she did for fun, and she stopped smiling.
"Things that are fun for me are not what other people consider
fun. If I'm at a party, that's torture. Like there was a big Junior
League gathering—"

I held up my hand. "Stop. *You* belong to the Junior League?"

She lifted one shoulder in a half shrug. "I know. It's weird. I
only like the service projects. I don't go to the social functions.
I don't talk on the phone because I don't have friends. Playing
on the computer, that's fun for me. I like going into stores and
looking at cosmetics counters and fragrances. But I do these
things completely alone."

As Lucy talked I made a mental checklist of her contradictions. She eschewed nail polish but had a manicure every week
to shape and buff her nails, minimized her own makeup but pored
over the latest beauty products online. She served the poor at
church but could not name them, joined the Junior League but
made no friends. She'd been married for more than twenty years,

yet didn't dare confront her husband. And although she'd soared through divinity school, she hadn't worked since. ("I could never be a minister because I'd never want to be in charge.")

"How does your husband feel about your giving up your career?"

"Oh, he's fine with it." She wrinkled her nose. "But then he's a workaholic."

"And how are you with that?"

"A couple of times I've actually suggested that he take a break, calm down, don't get all wrapped up in it. But he'll say, 'You are the last person to give me advice.' And I'm not a shining example. So I try to contain myself."

I pointed out the irony of a woman with a history of anorexia making that statement.

Lucy sipped her water. We'd finished eating. She glanced at her empty plate with a look of resignation. "Even now, much as I like to think of myself as completely over this, whenever I get upset, the first thought that pops into my head is, if I lose some weight I'll feel better. It's so superficial and so awful, but I still have that in me. I don't act on it, but I think it."

"The anorexic response is timeless," historian Rudolph Bell wrote in *Holy Anorexia*. Even in the Middle Ages, when saints like Catherine of Siena, Veronica Giuliani, and Clare of Assisi were claiming that starvation lifted them closer to God, what they were really seeking, according to Bell, was escape from the conflicts of daily life. "The medieval Italian girl striving for autonomy, not unlike the modern American, British, or Japanese girl faced with the same dilemma, sometimes shifted the contest from an outer world in which she faced seemingly sure defeat to an inner struggle to achieve mastery over herself, over her bodily urges." This certainly did sound like Lucy Romanello, and yet both Lucy's "anorexic response" and the saints' struck notably different chords than Candace's, Yvonne's, Ella Olds—or, for that matter, my own.

The four of us had felt miserable in the isolation of our eating disorder. As students we compulsively produced good grades even in classes we hated. Although uncomfortable in the spotlight, we could be counted on to perform. And, perhaps most crucially, we hoped by returning to health to become more connected with the world at large, not to pull back into ourselves. Lucy, like Kim Olensky, performed for her parents, teachers, bosses, and husband only up to a point. If challenged or criticized, she withdrew. It seemed to me that Lucy and Kim fit the anorexic profile that researchers Drew Westen and Jennifer Harnden-Fischer had dubbed overcontrolled. The personality type that psychologists most often associate with this profile is called, appropriately, avoidant.

Researchers estimate that as many as a third of restricting anorexics have avoidant personalities. Like people with obsessive-compulsive personalities, this group tends to be perfectionistic, but they are often more emotionally and sexually inhibited, more sensitive to criticism and shame, and more introverted. The avoidant view of perfection has less to do with rules, grades, or numbers on a scale than with a kind of transcendent or mystical love. To be perfect, to this way of thinking, is to be trouble free. In effect, invisible.

"The dizzy rapture of starving" is how Kathryn Harrison in her memoir *The Kiss* described her vision of anorexic perfection. "The power of needing nothing. By force of will I make myself the impossible sprite who lives on air, on water, on purity. It isn't just appetite for food that I deny, it's all appetite, all desire." Caroline Knapp's drill in *Appetites* was less rapturous but no less absolute: "Your needs are overwhelming? You can't depend on yourself or others to meet them? You don't even know what they are? Then need nothing."

Nothing in the realm of avoidance is not a Zen sort of nothing—not zero as meditative calm. Instead, it implies anxious negation: no risk, no love, no honesty, no wisdom, no fun, and ultimately no sensation at all. Significantly, however, it does not signify an absence of want. The want among these ascetics is usually voracious but so formless and inverted that few can even begin to describe it. That's because, as more than one psychologist described the problem to me, these anorexics feel "self less." It's a matter less of low self-esteem than no self at all.

In *The Spiral Staircase* Karen Armstrong recalled this self-lessness as a state that had been actively encouraged during her seven years in the convent but which propelled her into anorexia when she tried to function in the outside world. What she desperately, if inchoately, was expressing was her longing to recover a sense of herself as a whole and authentic individual. "What was the point of feeding my body when my mind and heart had been irreparably broken? And yet, in a way, I also felt that by starving myself I was reaching out to the world. I was asking for help. People kept telling me that I was fine and congratulating me on how well I was doing. But I was not fine and I wanted people to know this. . . . Look, I was saying, this is what I really feel like. Please notice."

"I remember often feeling that I didn't deserve, wasn't worthy of things," one former anorexic told me. "Money, treats, pretty clothes, or the same goodies that my sister got. This feeling was at the core of me." Asked about childhood dreams, another woman reflected, "I can't really remember having any." Or, as one of the subjects in psychologist Sheila Reindl's study of bulimia put it: "I don't even know how I feel . . . how to identify what I want."

Psychologists through most of the twentieth century assumed that such feelings of existential anomie resulted from faulty parenting. Often a pretty good case could be made against parents who abused or neglected or shamed their children into denying their true feelings. Karen Armstrong makes a similar case against her Catholic mothers when she writes of the frequency with which anorexia occurred in her convent. Three young nuns, including Karen, developed the eating disorder within months of other—and not because they were imitating supermodels. bodies had rebelled against the religious regime we had endured," Armstrong concludes. "I had been instructed by my superiors to subjugate my body to my will." But the prevalence of certain key traits among anorexics with no history of abuse or subjugation has made some psychiatrists question the wisdom of automatically or exclusively blaming outside forces. In the past few years researchers have been exploring other possible explanations for why some people seem naturally inclined to enjoy themselves, even under duress, while others seem intent on denying their very existence. What this research has shown is that pleasure, like perfectionism, plays an enormous role in eating disorders—and the way we do or don't process pleasure is largely a function of biology.

"Things that are fun for me are not what other people would typically consider fun." As I tried to make sense of Lucy's story in the context of others I'd heard, I imagined a continuum, with gregarious, fun-loving revelers at one end and monks who had taken a vow of silence at the other. Lucy and Kim Olensky, I suspected, would choose to plant themselves close to the monks. Ella, Yvonne, and I would probably gravitate more toward the middle. Picturing the continuum forced me to see, however, that our differences were not as great as I'd assumed. Those of us with obsessive-compulsive personalities might not be as shy or retiring as those who would qualify as avoidant, but at best we had a cautious relationship with pleasure. You weren't likely to find us at Mardi Gras (translation: Fat Tuesday), nor could we even approach the league of my sister-in-law, Mary.

"Oh, I *am* a hedonist!" Mary recently cried, swooning over a pair of well-braised short ribs. One of her life's dreams, she told me, is to dine at Napa Valley's five-star restaurant the French Laundry. Her pleasures include sailing in a beam reach with a steady six-knot wind in Pamet Sound off Cape Cod, drinking vintage cabernet with her girlfriends from college, receiving a foot rub, wrestling with her dog, and discovering really clever gizmos at tag sales. Ten years ago, Mary quit her corporate career to become a toy inventor, working from home, which means that she can, and often does, throw a dinner party on an hour's notice. Eating to her is one of life's many delights— never, ever, a problem

I marvel at such capacity for joy. I envy it, and I suspect I can identify with it more than Lucy or Kim might, but that is not to say I come to it naturally or easily. Not in such a sensuous way. And not with such abandon. I tend to think and see my way to-ward pleasure instead of touching or tasting it. Also, my enjoy-ment comes less from taking in sensation than from producing reflections of it. The milky light of winter, a man and his small child holding hands in silhouette against the ocean, the dark blizzard of crows that recently churned the sky outside my of-fice—such impressions excite me with the desire to turn them into something else: a phrase or picture or story. I find this process of creativity genuinely rewarding. However, the con-stant need to capture and take control of experience interferes with the immediacy and scope of feeling. I have to consciously remind myself to *stop* thinking; to absorb the light, shape, sound, texture, and smell of the moment; and let these sensa-tions happen to me instead of trying to take possession of them. This is the only effective way I've found to counter the sense I've had my whole life of being an observer rather than a par-ticipant—of witnessing the world through that "odd distance" that Marya Hornbacher likened to a wall of glass.

An important key to understanding this distance may lie in the fact that more than half of all anorexics and bulimics qual-ify as *alexithymic*: either they cannot accurately read or express their feelings, or they censor themselves so harshly that percep-tion becomes distorted. This is why Sheila Reindl titled her 2001 study of recovery from bulimia *Sensing the Self*. "And here," she wrote, "the word *sense* is as important as the word *self*." Reindl concluded that to overcome an eating disorder one must literally relearn how to feel through touch, taste, smell, sound. How much sweetness, how much warmth, how much size is "just right"? Reindl's subjects, like Goldilocks, "'came to their senses' and learned to trust their sensed experience, in particular their sense of 'enoughness.'"

Karen Armstrong recalled her own "first flicker of true recovery" while listening to a recitation of T. S. Eliot's poem "Ash-Wednesday," a serene meditation on releasing the past in order to cultivate new joy. "My appreciation was no longer wholly cerebral. It was an essentially emotional, intuitive response that somehow involved my entire personality, reaching something deeply embedded within. I had thought I had lost this capacity forever, but here it was again. There was a complete and satisfying fit between my inner and outer worlds." Sensation is the opposite of numbness and denial. To experience sensation means making contact, allowing closeness, and letting go of inhibition.

But this is a tall order for people who instinctively pull away from or intellectualize emotional and sensory contact. "Appetites," Harvard psychiatrist David Herzog told me, "are scary for them. Emotions must be tightly controlled. To do that, my anorexic patients in particular convince themselves emotions are unnecessary. *I don't need anger. I don't need delight.*" Herzog, along with researchers Eugene Beresin and Christopher Gordon, published a landmark study in 1989 that looked at the subjective experience of recovery from anorexia nervosa. That research expanded into an ongoing longitudinal study, tracking more than two hundred individuals who were first treated for anorexia or bulimia between 1987 and 1991. Herzog told me about one woman who was so disconnected from her body that she was in her seventh month before she knew she was pregnant. She's now in her mid-twenties and physically both she and her son are healthy, but Herzog still sees the woman in therapy. Her current challenge is to achieve intimacy with her child. "The fear is that sensation will overwhelm her."

Similar observations led Walter Kaye to doubt the theory he'd learned early in his clinical training that the sensory discomfort that accompanies anorexia was caused by an inability to fully or automatically experience physical pleasure. Given the way his patients flinched and drew back from stimulation as varied as being touched, the smell of bacon, or the sound of Beethoven's music, Kaye suspected that for people with anorexia, the problem might actually be *too much* pleasure—chemically speaking.

The key to pleasure in the human brain is dopamine, a neurotransmitter that influences movement, desire, appetite, memory, and problem solving. It also helps determine when we are sated or satisfied—when we've had enough not only of food but of touch, smell, talk, or other stimulation. So in 2005, Kaye and his colleague Guido Frank used positron emission tomography imaging (PET scans) to watch the activity of receptors that bind dopamine in the brain. People who had a history of restricting anorexia (all were of normal weight and at least one year recovered) showed a much more active response to dopamine than did healthy women with no history of eating disorders. By contrast, other researchers have found unusually *low* dopamine receptor activity in the brains of the obese, as well as in compulsive gamblers and substance abusers. The researchers are still sorting out exactly how these results fit together, but one possibility is that their hyperactive response causes people with anorexia to be so overwhelmed by dopamine during sensory overload that what feels good to most people, to them feels bad. Instead of enjoying typical sources of pleasure, they find relief in numbness. This might explain why a surprise party, which would delight most of her fellow Junior Leaguers, would be a form of torture to Lucy Romanello, and why Lucy's ideas of fun (taking a solitary walk, going to church, reading a book, listening to sacred music) all safely contain and control the level of stimulation she is exposed to.

The pleasure principle could also help to explain the ambivalent relationship so many people with eating disorders have with achievement, fame, and fortune—what American culture promotes as "success." Again, Lucy may be an extreme example, having excelled in school and on the job, only to retreat into self-imposed obscurity; but I was not, as Lucy might say, a shining example, either. I was the one who sabotaged a modeling career by losing too much weight and went on to squander most of my time at Yale in hiding. I thought I wanted to succeed, but obviously something didn't feel right. Peter Kramer explains in *Listening to Prozac* that people who can't fully experience pleasure do not, in fact, feel the same thrill that others do when they ace an exam or get a promotion or see their name in lights. As Audrey Hepburn reflected on her first critical Broadway success, her starring role as *Ondine* in 1954: "It's like reaching an important birthday and finding you're exactly the same. All I feel is the responsibility to live up to it. And even, with luck, survive it." Hepburn lost ten pounds during rehearsals for *Ondine*, had to be force-fed through its run, and within months had quit the show and withdrawn into isolation as her weight continued to plummet.

The problem is that we are told so insistently—at home, in school, on television, at the movies—that we *should* succeed that many of us start to obey this rule without thinking. Minus pleasure, the result can be what Judith Viorst in *Imperfect Control* calls "pathological persistence." Example: Lucy spent eighteen years working at a job she loathed, never requesting a transfer, never attempting another career, until she was so desperate for relief she quit working altogether. One can say this was a free choice, but a case could also be made that it was only as free as the playing of a pianist with a gun pointed at her head. To escape the gun requires either a tolerance for risk, the exact opposite of an avoidant trait, or a sense of intolerable desperation.

Irene Slocum began to feel that desperation in 1966, when she entered seventh grade in Portland, Oregon. Irene read poetry and wore moccasins and didn't know how to make friends. When the other girls talked about who was wearing whose ID bracelet or which couples had just broken up, Irene couldn't think what to say. Girls, she could see, were supposed to have fun. But what about girls like her, who didn't *feel* fun—or didn't feel it the way other girls seemed to? It made Irene nervous to be around these girls, especially in the school cafeteria, amid the high-pitched laughter and glittering trays full of food, so she spent her lunch breaks in vacant classrooms, reading instead of eating. By ninth grade she'd dropped from 120 to 80 pounds. The next year, she dropped out of school.

Irene was fifty-two when we first met, at a writers' conference where she was working on a memoir about her life in the rural West. She was still wiry thin and excruciatingly shy, yet when she learned about the book I was writing she asked me up to her room in the dorms where we were staying, poured us each a cup of Bailey's Irish Cream, and talked as if she'd been waiting her whole life for someone to ask her who she was.

"I threw tantrums as a little kid," she said with a smile. "I remember my father carrying me away from the dinner table, up the stairs, and I would claw the family portraits off the wall as we passed." Her parents were "bookish," she said, her father an engineer and her mother a teacher. Their silence scared her. "I knew I was different, and I knew that was not okay." But she didn't know how she was different or what she wanted. She felt trapped, both at home and at school.

After she quit high school, her parents searched for somewhere to send her away, and Irene did not object. They agreed on a farm school in Vermont. "I loved the place, the community, the sense that the students were connected. We grew our own food, prepared all our meals, tended chickens and cows, tapped maples. We also made things—cabinets, pots." She learned to have friends. And she ate. "The farm may not have been good for everyone, but it was good for me."

Irene told me she still grows vegetables, still makes furniture as well as teapots, masks, and her own clothes. But the farm is not the only reason she regained her health. If it were that simple, she said, her sister would have recovered, too. Like Irene, her older sister, Eleanor, is "very, very sensitive. The slightest hint of teasing will make her cry." Also like Irene, Eleanor became anorexic, though not until she went away to college. Eleanor, too, retreated to the country, marrying young as Irene had and living off the grid. "But Eleanor's husband was a fanatic." Irene shook her head. "He built their house himself, wouldn't have electricity or plumbing. She had to fetch their water from the well down the hill, so she was carrying these thirty-pound buckets twice a day—"

I asked how much Eleanor herself weighed.

"About eighty pounds. A big part of Eleanor's problem is that she never could gain the courage to leave her husband, even though he treated her like his slave. The other part was that, because of the anorexia, she couldn't have kids. They adopted a little girl, which got her enough outside herself to stay alive, but she's still not really recovered."

I tasted the thick sweet, liquored cream Irene had served me. This was not a drink either of us would have touched thirty years earlier. Irene swallowed a big gulp and smiled. "What really saved me were my kids."

Irene was unusual among the women I interviewed in that she married before she was twenty—and had four children. "I didn't know what I was doing," she said. "I didn't think I had a choice. But it turned out they were real in a way that nothing else in my life was. They taught me to play. We'd dance and sing and draw. We had dogs and rabbits." She grinned. "We made messes together."

I tried to picture Irene as the radiant young mother she must once have been—safe in the company of her children. But the downside of marrying so young, for her, was that she didn't love her husband, and that unhappiness marked her in ways that were impossible to overlook. "I had to be strong for the kids," she said when I asked about the marriage, "but my husband was so much my opposite. He was a lawyer, very social. He always wanted to entertain, to join this club and that club. He never stopped *talking*." She said this as another ex-wife might complain of her spouse's abuse, but I understood that for Irene this barrage of noise did feel like a kind of abuse.

"I couldn't be strong around him. I just wanted to curl up into a ball, to get away," she said. "It wasn't his fault. He thought he loved me. I felt so guilty, I asked for nothing when I left the marriage. But he had his next wife all lined up as soon as I was out the door, and she was one of those starched and pressed women who could hardly wait to throw a cocktail party." Irene pushed a hand through her wild mane of hair. "Anyway, I learned to survive poverty, and that made me tough."

She moved into a trailer on a rented plot of rural land and worked as an aide in a home for schizophrenics, for whom she felt an instinctive empathy. All the skills she'd learned in that farm school now became tools for survival. Late in her forties she married a Nepalese potter who practiced Buddhism and spoke little English. "We communicate a lot through silence." The fine web of lines around her eyes crinkled as she smiled.

It was late and time to go, but I was curious about Irene's children. "How did your kids do with all these changes? How did they handle adolescence?"

"Oh, they were fine. One of my sons graduated from Princeton and the other from Reed. My eldest daughter is in graduate school at Stanford now, and the younger one just got out of Oberlin." Irene gave her drink a thoughtful sip. "You know, looking back, I think there were people in high school who could have been my friends. There were always people in my life who cared about me. I just couldn't get out of my own head. I was too busy running away."

I think Irene is too hard on her younger self. As psychoanalyst Erich Fromm wrote in *To Have or to Be?*: "We internalize the authoritarian structure of our society," and most of us, depending on our class and social position, learn early that we are expected to get a particular kind of education, get married at a particular time of life, get a particular kind of job, and ultimately get as rich and famous as our circumstances will allow. If we are female, we are also trained to hunger for a better face and body. But all this getting rarely gains us a sense of our own identity. "Most people," according to Fromm, "believe they are following their own will and are unaware that their will itself is conditioned and manipulated." In other words, they operate under an illusion of decisiveness without actually being self-directed. For those, like Irene, who do sense and recoil from this manipulation, the need to feel real may demand physical as well as emotional relocation, to a different kind of community or culture.

The true existential choice, Fromm wrote, is not between wanting this or that—miniskirts or boyfriends, money or love— but between wanting to claim possession of things, roles, and even relationships (*Let me have*) and wanting to freely exist, express oneself, give, and experience (*Let me be*). "Everything and anything can become an object of craving: things we use in daily life, property, rituals, good deeds, knowledge, and thoughts." Even abstinence can become an object of craving, which is why wanting nothing is so unsatisfying: "In the very attempt to suppress having and consuming, the person may be equally preoccupied with having and consuming." What do the medieval starving saints, Karen Carpenter, Caroline Knapp, and Mary-Kate Olsen all have in common? An all-consuming compulsion to avoid consuming.

The wisdom Irene had achieved by learning to farm and in raising her children was more in line with Buddha's: "When I am hungry, I eat; when I am thirsty, I drink." Respect the needs of the human body as well as the human soul. Savor food as you savor life. Irene had hardly become a hedonist; that was not in her makeup. But she had managed to create a full, rich life on her own terms—incorporating her shyness and anxieties and respecting them instead of trying to deny them (as she would have had to in order to stay with her first husband). Contrast this with the attitude of so many others with a history of anorexia or bulimia: *The more I suffer, the better I am; the less I suffer, the worse I am.* Or, as Lucy Romanello admitted, "The thought patterns about thinness—about how much I'm eating, what I'm eating, whether I'll feel guilty afterward—are always there at the back of my mind." What would Buddha say?

He might well ask, Why *guilt*? Or, Why *fear*? Eating too much can cause physical discomfort, and we might rationally regret eating extra calories that we'll later have to burn off or accept as an added ounce of flesh. But how does eating a chocolate-chip cookie become a moral issue? When I was fourteen I used the nightly television images of children starving during the Biafran famine as an excuse to starve myself. If I cannot save them, I thought, at least let me not consume the food that might have saved them. My self-imposed hunger, of course, left me so listless and self-obsessed I never considered participating in the many relief efforts that were making a real difference in Biafra. Years later, when working as a flight attendant, I thought of this paradox every time I demonstrated the use of oxygen masks: "Parents, place the mask over your own face and mouth *first*, so you can then assist your children." Analysis of past airline disasters had taught United that self-sacrifice typically hurt more people than it helped. But anorexic thinking is predicated on self-sacrifice.

In London, Janet Treasure has found that such thinking can actually be mapped. Using a method called functional magnetic resonance imaging (fMRI), Treasure's group at the Maudsley Hospital has watched the brain "in action" as it responds to images of food. What they've found is that in people with no history of eating disorders, the sight of a strawberry cheesecake, say, will excite the lateral region of the brain normally responsible for appetite. But with anorexia and bulimia, the dominant response to food comes from a region at the front of the brain normally involved in making decisions and regulating anxiety. The longer a person has been ill, the stronger the response of this frontal region, which also dispenses moral judgment such as guilt. When people return to normal eating habits, however, *multiple* areas of the brain spring into action to override the disordered response to food. This patching, Treasure said, acts as a brake on the impulse to suppress appetite. The more time that passes without relapse, the stronger and more permanent the patch becomes. It cannot, however, produce a truly normal appetite response. Even decades after their last fast or purge, former anorexics and bulimics will respond to the sight of a layer cake with a complex mix of attraction, resistance, guilt, calculation, permission, and release.

The good news in this research is that the brain appears to constantly rebuild itself, allowing the mind to gradually gain control over even entrenched afflictions. So, while Lucy Romanello still wrestled with occasional residual feelings of disgust about food, she now accepted that roast beef was a source of health rather than guilt or fear. And while Irene Slocum might not attack her meals with the same gustatory pleasure as my schoolmates Lia and Jen, she could associate a cupcake with the pleasure she had baking with her kids or a loaf of bread with the memory of kneading dough at that farm in Vermont. These connections helped her to enjoy eating. Health requires the conscious, year-in-and-year-out cultivation of just such satisfying connections.

When I began to emerge from anorexia, I knew that I wanted, as Irene put it, to feel real. What I did *not* want was nothing. But after suppressing my feelings for so long, how was I to act on them? The first step, I discovered quite accidentally, was to explore joy.

Even now, I wince at this word. The concept of joy has been taken hostage by Christmas carols and perfume manufacturers, turned, like so much in our culture, into a merchandising slogan. Moreover, joy has dubious meaning for someone who has difficulty sensing pleasure. But joy is not the same as pleasure. It is both more variable and more profound. "Joy," Fromm wrote, "is not the ecstatic fire of the moment. Joy is the glow that accompanies being." When we feel joy, we feel that we are growing and fully alive, and in this higher zone of desire, pleasure has new meaning.

As a painting major I spent most of my college days in the studio among graduate art students. Unlike most undergraduate Yalies of the seventies, who had learned at prep school to create the illusion of joy through marijuana, LSD, all-night games of bridge, and keg parties, these older artists came mostly from blue-collar backgrounds in Philadelphia, Yonkers, and Brooklyn; and they relied on art as their lifeline. Peter, for example, was a short, ambitious Greek American who made abstract expressionist paintings so large he required a scaffold to finish them. Louisa wrinkled her nose when she laughed and crafted jewel-colored assemblages that looked like toys. Dean chain-smoked and painted large, amorphous abstracts with one arm because he'd lost the other to a farm machine in his teens. Denise talked tough about her personal bankruptcy and made paintings of the box-shaped tract houses where she'd grown up. And then there was Marjorie, an ample blond who dressed like a trucker and painted herself nude surrounded by cakes, doughnuts, cookies—who laid her hunger out on canvas in a way that at once mortified and instructed me. Marjorie and the others were not perfect, not rich, not paragons of beauty or fashion—nor did they aspire to be. Many carried core traumas and losses, but they worked these out through their art, and in so doing managed a kind of exuberance, a letting go that I had never seen before. They filled their studios with jazz and color. They ate with gusto. And they loved to dance.

Every week the MFA students threw a party in the large main floor gallery of the Art & Architecture Building. Technically, these were openings for the shows of student artwork that rotated on the gallery walls throughout the year, but their practical purpose was fun. Fun was then, for me, a foreign concept. Up until my first graduate opening, I associated parties with the make-out sessions I'd avoided in high school or the dark, beer-soaked undergraduate mixers that throbbed across campus each weekend. But at the gallery openings the lights stayed on. There were no cliques, no social intrigues. I knew and trusted everyone in the room. This minimized the sexual heat and freed even me to dance.

I was about as adept at dancing as I was at fun. No one as uncomfortable in her skin as I was could possibly dance well. But at these A&A openings nobody was a particularly great dancer. People moved solo. They danced in groups. They traded partners in square-dance formations, swinging and shimmying and laughing. Nobody showed off. And nobody stood awkwardly on the sidelines.

The music—headlined by the Supremes, the Four Tops, Gladys Knight, the Temptations—was key. Unlike the music of the Rolling Stones, which dominated the campus mixers and which seemed intent on assault, Motown had a sweetness and rhythm that lifted me to my feet. There was joy in the notes and joy in our dancing, and the enduring lesson for me was that this joy had no strings attached. To feel this happy I didn't have to eat or not eat. I didn't have to perform. I didn't have to suffer or pay the price later. I didn't have to pretend. Every week, for those few hours, I could safely play.

Here was a crucial lesson for gaining health: wanting for nothing can simply mean wanting to enjoy being alive. That kind of being involves all the senses, all the emotions. It opens us to the world, to feel the warmth of the sun, the cool breeze play across our skin. It fills us with the desire to kiss those we love. It inspires us to devour the beauty created by Vermeer and Bach. It propels us to dance. These free and limitless pleasures are the delicacies that satisfy our deepest hungers. We deny these hungers at our peril.

5

GOOD BAD GIRLS
Shame

She failed, and I must destroy her. Obliterate
this good daughter with one so bad that what
she does is unspeakable.
—Kathryn Harrison, *The Kiss*

HANNAH WINTERS AS A CHILD was her mother's favorite, the
baby of six. She earned straight A's. She also drank beer and
smoked dope at age twelve—because some older kids told her
to. In college she joined her mother's sorority, took ballet three
times a week, and decided to stop eating. "I had no sense of
what was normal," she recalled twenty years later. "I remember
running ten miles, then bingeing, giving blood, lying about my
weight. I'd go to the grocery store, write bad checks for the
food, then sneak around to gas stations to throw up."

Hannah made a striking contrast to the women I'd interviewed to that point. Now forty-two, mother of two little girls,
and a hospital administrator in rural Iowa, she remembers herself as neither avoidant nor perfectionistic but as eager growing
up. "I was outgoing, and when I was little I was desperate to
please." She was also impulsive, a trait especially common

among "undercontrolled" bulimics and anorexics wh
tiple methods to purge.

We usually think of impulses as things we *want* to do—call a
friend, eat a peach, make love—and compulsions as things we
feel we *must* do—make more money, confess, be polite to our
in-laws. Psychologists, however, reserve the label *impulse* for behavior that is volatile, spontaneous, and potentially harmful.
Shoplifting is an impulse. So is playing Russian roulette. *Compulsive* behavior, by contrast, is driven by obsessively fearful
thoughts and is meant, if superstitiously, to avoid harm. Checking over and over to make sure the car door is locked, avoiding
the cracks in the sidewalk to protect your mother's back—these
are compulsions.

Psychologists used to consider compulsive and impulsive disorders to be polar opposites and therefore mutually exclusive. In
the 1990s that view began to change. The new research on
serotonin and the success of SSRIs such as Prozac in treating
both bulimia and OCD suggested that similar imbalances of
neurotransmitters in the brain can produce a range of behaviors. Researchers at Canada's McGill University reported in
2004 that bulimics and binge-purge anorexics could be divided
into two groups according to the activity of serotonin in their
brains. The majority of bingers and purgers in this five-year
study showed consistently low levels of serotonin density and
activity, both during and after their eating disorder. But another
smaller group instead had *high* serotonin function.

The women who had low serotonin tended, like the young
Hannah Winters, to be impulsive and emotionally erratic. In
addition to bingeing and purging, many engaged in cutting,
drinking, drug use, reckless driving, and sexual promiscuity.
Many fit the description for borderline personality disorder
(BPD), a condition that, objectively, seems the opposite of
obsessive-compulsive personality disorder.

Whereas obsessive-compulsive traits tend to suppress impulses, most borderline traits heighten impulsiveness, often with destructive consequences. *I Hate You, Don't Leave Me*, the title of a popular book about BPD by psychiatrist Jerold Kreisman and Hal Straus, sums up both the behavior and the inner conflict of the disorder. "A pervasive pattern of instability of mood, interpersonal relationships, and self-image," is how the diagnostic manual describes BPD. "Promiscuous sex with more partners than I could count or remember," is how Rachel Reiland recalled her behavior in *Get Me Out of Here*, her memoir of BPD, "heavy drinking and illegal drug use that had slowed with the births of [her children] but were still present. Midnight runs . . . anorexia . . . I'd never made a bona fide suicide attempt, never swallowed pills or put a gun to my head, but I'd thought about it plenty and talked about it frequently." Seventy percent of borderlines make suicide attempts. And 70 percent have a history of physical, sexual, or emotional abuse as children. These numbers almost exactly matched the rates of suicidal behavior and childhood abuse among the low-serotonin bulimics in the McGill study.

The women with *high* serotonin in the study were by contrast both obsessive and compulsive, and few had experienced any kind of childhood abuse. Temperamentally, they seemed to resemble restricting anorexics. But in fact, the two types of bulimics had more in common than not. Both showed higher levels of impulsive behavior than either the restrictors or women with no eating disorder.

Imagine a child on a swing whose feet don't touch the ground. Her impulses push her forward; her compulsions push her back. She can scream, "Enough!" all she likes, but she doesn't know how to stop. Now multiply the swings and picture them all going at once. That gives you some idea what happens inside the brain. Impulses and compulsions don't take turns, and no one has just one or the other. A child throwing a tantrum because she can't have a cookie, clinging to her mother even as she screams at her, is in that moment drowning in contradictory impulses and compulsions. A healthy child, with the help of understanding parents and normal brain chemistry, learns to manage these colliding waves of need and urgency as she grows up, resisting destructive impulses and yielding to healthy desires; moderating compulsions; and balancing spontaneity, reflection, and delayed gratification. Most of us consider this kind of emotional management to be a sign of maturity. Disorders like bulimia and BPD, however, indicate this management system either hasn't developed properly or has broken down.

But the chemistry of serotonin answers only part of the mystery. Lisa Lilenfeld, who worked with Walter Kaye on some of the first studies of serotonin's role in eating disorders, says that while her research strongly suggests that self-injuring bulimics have "some kind of deficiency or something in their serotonin receptors that's not quite what the average person has, there are lots of people walking around with deficient serotonin systems that aren't cutting their arm and throwing up. People learn other coping behaviors. Good or bad self-esteem makes a difference."

Sheila Reindl agrees. Her research convinced her that with bulimia, the individual usually has a strong sense of her true nature but "feels she must hide the most intense aspects of herself because they will be judged or shunned by others." Typically, Reindl found, this feeling is based on experience, or a series of experiences, dating from early childhood.

"My mom raced stock cars," Hannah told me during the first of our phone interviews. "She is a hoot. But from infancy I got the message that my job was to make her happy. We shopped together. We binged on candy together when I was little. We dieted together when I was a teenager. Once she told me, 'You know, Hannah, I thought after five kids I'd finally come up with the perfect concoction of child.' " But Hannah's weight at that point had dropped below 90 pounds. Her mother finished her thought: "Now I see I was wrong."

Most of Hannah's siblings were world-beaters. Her four older brothers organized peace rallies, built model rockets, dated homecoming queens, and graduated Phi Beta Kappa. (One married a Yale classmate of mine, who had prompted Hannah to contact me.) Her older sister was more complicated. Like Hannah, she suffered from depression and occasional panic attacks. Yet only Hannah developed an eating disorder.

It began during her freshman year at UCLA. "I was rooming with an upperclassman. And I was in body-beautiful, face-beautiful Southern California." Hannah then, as she is again in her forties, was plump, with Shirley Temple curls and a heart-shaped face that belonged to another era. She had grown up in Des Moines. In LA she felt invisible. "I remember writing in my journal—a rather corny statement, but it was the truth—'A *seed of sorrow has been planted in my heart.*' I was in a women's center group-therapy session, and suddenly the room started to have a different color. Like I only saw people's auras. I was trying to explain how I felt, but they weren't getting it. Afterward, I remember walking over a little bridge and making the decision that I was going to stop eating."

Just like that. A simple impulse to place one goal above all others, making everything else insignificant by comparison. Compulsion followed. "I was five foot three, a hundred thirty pounds, and dropped to one hundred seven; then one hundred was my goal. Then anything under one hundred." Hannah's father, who was an internist, and her psychiatrist both urged her to be hospitalized. Unfortunately, the hospital they selected didn't specialize in eating disorders, and after just a month her insurance ran out. "After I went back to school, I remember one night, standing outside in the rain. I had gone to an Overeaters Anonymous meeting, and I was this skinny little girl among all these fat ladies. All I heard them say was, I will have this disease for the rest of my life. That did it. I stood by the roadside watching the cars go by, imagining myself jumping in front of them. The next morning I told my psychiatrist, and he put me back in the hospital."

But she still wasn't working with doctors who understood eating disorders. "They let me out on a pass, and instead of going to class I went straight to the grocery store and stole and ate cookies and drank a diet Dr Pepper, and went upstairs to the bathroom to throw up . . . and I got caught. They took me to the police station, had mug shots taken, the whole deal. I started sobbing."

Back in the hospital Hannah was put on seventy-two-hour hold. "I remember my mother visiting me, and she had gained twenty pounds through this ordeal, just wondering what she did wrong." Hannah's feelings of responsibility for her mother kicked in. She finished out the school year, but her grade point average was now in steady decline, her bulimia unchecked. She transferred to Pitzer, a smaller college where she felt less anonymous, and joined the cross-country team. Every morning she ran ten miles. After just two months, she had another breakdown.

"I'd gone to Commons and got a huge amount of food, and I threw it up. Then I had a test in statistics, and I didn't do very well. And I'd just broken up with my boyfriend. I was lying there on the quad and feeling like such a failure. Changing to a new college wasn't going to make a difference. I was never going to be free of this obsession with my body being thin and with food." She went back to her dorm room and overdosed on sedatives.

Incredibly, no one noticed. Even after she woke up two days later, "Nobody really got it that I'd made a major suicide attempt." No one was going to rescue her. Not her boyfriend. Not her parents. Not her friends or her sister. "I started meeting with a new counselor, and she said, 'Look, you can get over this, but it's going to take two years for the behavior to stop.'

"I started by just making myself keep the food in. I'd be really full, and I was gaining weight, and I'd think I could throw this up, but, no, I told someone I was going to stop by their dorm room and I have a test tomorrow and I really want to study because I'm doing pretty well in this class. I started choosing normalcy."

It was a false start, however. Hannah could will herself to moderate her eating and stop purging. She could, and did, graduate. She moved to a small town and supported herself with a clerical job. But none of that corrected the chemical regulation of her brain. She continued to drink and smoke dope, then would stop cold turkey—and begin again, heavily. A fainting disorder eventually replaced her eating disorder. "I would just shut down. A couple of times I stopped breathing." At twenty-six Hannah was back in the hospital.

This particular hospital's chief of staff was a bulky, take-charge man her father's age, who had met Hannah a few weeks earlier at a local bar. He assigned himself to her case and included a breast exam in his initial examination. "Later, he said, 'I was really enjoying that breast exam.' Then he kissed me." Stunned, Hannah went along with him. "But one day somebody in my group-therapy session talked about their sexual addiction—and that description of their history of acting out struck me. I tried to stop the affair, but he wouldn't believe I wanted to end it, and not even my therapist believed me when I tried to report him. Suddenly I felt trapped. I went into the bathroom, took down a lightbulb, rolled it in a towel, and broke it. I had once before cut my arm when I was twenty-five, but this time when I started cutting my neck and my arm I wasn't able to numb out. I started screaming because I didn't want to be in pain physically. I wanted help."

Hannah phoned her mother. Her father came for her. "They took my dad into a room and said, 'She's very manipulative. She's dangerous.' He brought me home and took me to a psychologist he trusted, who said, 'She's not psychotic; she has borderline personality disorder.'"

Hannah was treated with behavioral and cognitive therapy, antidepressants, antianxiety medications, and psychoanalysis. Finally she began to recover.

"What I realize now," Hannah told me, "is how easy it was to cross the line, to put myself in situations where somebody was behaving toward me in a way that would lead to something terrible, but I didn't feel I had the voice to stop it." Her subsequent years in treatment taught her to be profoundly respectful of the mind's sensitivity to experience, especially during childhood. She remembered an incident when she was fifteen and visiting her aunt. "This man—her company—came into the bedroom. I think he thought he'd find my aunt but he found me there, and he started to get my panties off and was touching me all over." Hannah didn't like it, but she went along with him just as she later went along when her doctor seduced her. She'd also gone along with a babysitter who molested her when she was eight. Each time, Hannah recalled, "I felt as if something had died in me. It's that whole experience that parallels the denial of my body in self-starvation."

Psychoanalysis at last led her back to the event that most likely began this syndrome. "I was kidnapped when I was nine months old. We were living in Belgium, and my parents asked the housekeeper to watch me when they went away. Well, the housekeeper's daughter was a prostitute, and she and her boyfriend took off with me. Police were called, and it was kind of a big deal. It wasn't for ransom or anything, but they kept me for three days."

Trauma, at any age, produces anatomical changes in the brain, and even if these changes do not have an obvious effect on behavior, they still can shape our deepest responses to anxiety. A NIMH study conducted from the late 1980s into the 1990s tracked 186 girls, half of whom had been abused, to determine if biological changes were indeed a result of childhood sexual abuse. The abused girls were found to have abnormally high levels of testosterone, initially higher and later lower than normal levels of cortisol, increases in immune system abnormalities, and abnormal changes in the regulation of heart rate under stress. Another study in 1993 found that combat soldiers who had been physically or sexually abused as children were nearly four times more likely to suffer from post-traumatic stress disorder than soldiers from the same battles who had not been abused. According to psychiatrist Peter Kramer, people who have suffered serious early trauma have trouble later coping with losses and threats that others would consider minor. Eventually, Kramer writes, heightened sensitivity and fear become part of a person's everyday personality. This could explain why such a high percentage of women with borderline personality disorder are abuse survivors and why borderline traits can develop in people of any temperament. Studies have found that about 40 percent of patients hospitalized for bulimia or binge-purge anorexia also have borderline symptoms.

Things happen. Psychological disorders evolve not through the smooth coalescence of genetics and family and culture but in reaction to shocks along the way. Identical twins may be raised as a single unit in the same family. Both have the same vulnerable temperament, yet only one twin develops anorexia. Why? Because certain experiences—what researchers call "unique environmental effects"—have affected her that didn't happen to her sister. Maybe she was injured during birth. Maybe she was fed second as a baby and never got enough. Maybe she fell and hit her head while learning to walk. Maybe someone teased her about being too fat to take ballet. Maybe something worse.

As a young child I trusted my parents implicitly. I had no secrets, nor was I afraid to tell them what I thought. That changed when I was seven. Suddenly I kept my feelings to myself. I was happy to have my mother do the talking. I assumed this was normal, just as I would later assume my dieting was normal. But what had happened to change the way I related to my parents? Why the sudden shift to secrecy at that particular age? These, I now realize, are critical questions, yet even though I wrote the answer in *Solitaire* more than twenty years ago, the questions didn't occur to me until just recently.

Let's start, then, with the answer:

Thanksgiving 1960. It's the year the Jones boys slather their pumpkin pie with ketchup while our parents argue, over chestnut dressing and creamed onions, about the future of JFK. It's the year my brother and Chas Jones, both fifteen, remain downstairs after dinner with the grown-ups while Cliff Jones and his buddy Dick take me up to the attic. Aged twelve, they laugh. Aged seven, I don't.

I believe what they tell me: it's just fooling around. It's my privilege to be included in their games. One little girl with two big boys, I am their obedient slave, anxious to please as long as they let me stay. Oh, please, please like me! Please accept me! Show that you want me, that you approve. I'll do anything to prove that I'm good enough to belong in your club!

We play tag around the attic. Catching splinters in our socks and cobwebs in our hair, we sing about Casey Jones and choo-choo-choo through the dark, musty closets. Downstairs, the adults laugh, lean back, and groan with satiety. They think we're watching TV.

"I know! Let's take off our clothes and play horse!" Cliff whispers. Dick eagerly seconds the notion.

I keep quiet. You can play horse with your clothes on just as well. I have never seen a boy in the raw—or wanted to. I know what my mother would say if she knew. But the boys will like me if I do this, and how can I say no to them?

Cliff goes down to lock the door at the bottom of the stairs. Then we strip and play horse. They ride me bareback on their shoulders. They toss me back and forth while hushing my nervous shrieks. I am frightened but too scared to show it.

"Now let's switch places." Cliff and Dick giggle as they lead me to a corner under the eaves. Cliff lies on his back, knees bent, and stretches his arms to receive me. Dick lifts me over him and guides my movements from behind as I straddle Cliff's naked body. Crouch, kneel, stroke, stroke. Our skin sticks. It tickles and makes me queasy. This is not fun. Even the boys have stopped laughing. Their stiffened genitals disgust me as they graze my chest and belly, explore between my thighs and touch, poking the skin inside me. Not talking, the boys tickle me to keep smiling even as I long to pull loose and run. I feel like an animal.

When my father calls, it's time to go home, we scramble for our clothes. Cliff swears me to secrecy. I'm part of the club, but won't be if I tell. They needn't worry. Whatever it is we've done wrong, I know it's my fault. An adventure in the attic. I never said no.

I included this incident in *Solitaire* because it helped explain why I loathed my body as a child: I starved to desex myself. But now I realize that night in the attic had an even more profound effect on my connection to my parents. For weeks after the incident I was hounded by nightmares that tapped out an archetypal code. The one that repeated most frequently featured a witch like Margaret Hamilton in *The Wizard of Oz* chasing me in the dark around a glowing swimming pool that contained an electric eel. If I ran away from the pool the witch would catch me; if I jumped in the water the eel would electrocute me. So I kept running in Freudian circles until, in a panic, I woke. The first few times this happened I sought refuge in my mother's bed, but in spite of her welcoming softness, the nightmare would return. Again and again she failed to protect me. This was not my mother's fault. How could she save me from something she didn't even know had happened?

Nevertheless, after that, I kept more of my inner life secret from my parents. Without knowing why, I also began to engage in activities that were bizarrely at odds with my basic nature, that I knew to be "bad," yet that I seemed unable to control. Just a month after my evening in the attic, I stole downstairs at four o'clock on Christmas morning and methodically opened every present addressed to me. When my mother found me out, I registered her hurt and unhappiness and promised never to do it again, but I strangely felt no remorse. A few weeks later, I took my Barbie doll (a toy that my mother despised for its flagrant sexuality, but which I had insisted I wanted) to a hidden corner of the basement and used a pin to puncture nipples in her breasts and a vagina between her legs. The smoothness of her plastic skin bothered me, and the act of anatomically correcting her soothed something deep inside me. Afterward, I hid the doll in shame and never played with it again. That spring I entered a neighbor's house through an open window, pocketed a handful of change, a hole punch, and a pitch pipe that I was certain would never be missed. I told myself I was "just fooling around." Never caught, I was never forced to reveal my secrets and so kept hoarding more.

I binged for the first time when I was nine. Alone one afternoon, I sat watching *The Match Game*, eating Oreos, drinking Hawaiian Punch. I hated being alone, hated the fact that I lived in a neighborhood where I was the only child, hated the fact that whenever I visited a friend's house I felt like a trespasser. I stared at the television screen and methodically ate and drank. When I snapped out of my trance I'd eaten the entire three-tier package of Oreos and finished the pitcher of punch. I was still too young to fear that this would make me fat, but I knew that it was excessive, wrong, shameful. *Pathetic* was the word that came to mind as I shoved the empty package into the trash.

Good girls do bad things, according to Sheila Reindl (who credits D. W. Winnicott and Freud for the insight), in order to make sense of experiences they cannot emotionally comprehend. "Being unable to understand why one feels guilty is so unsettling that it can lead a person to do something bad so that she can at last attribute her guilt to a specific behavior." Scottish psychoanalyst W. R. D. Fairbairn explained such guilty bludgeoning this way: "It is better to be a sinner in a world ruled by God than to live in a world ruled by the Devil. A sinner in a world ruled by

God may be bad; but there is always a certain sense of security to be derived from the fact that the world around is good . . . there is always a hope of redemption. In a world ruled by the Devil . . . the only prospect is one of death and destruction."

I didn't know of anyone else who acted like I did until I was ten years old and saw the movie *Breakfast at Tiffany's*. Audrey Hepburn *was* for me Holly Golightly, the whisper-thin young woman who invents a glamorous persona at odds with her shameful childhood, who climbs in and out of windows, shoplifts, stays up all night, suffers fits of fear and sadness that she disguises with convincing sophistication, and mistrusts love and intimacy so that she cultivates "rats" for suitors even as she flees those who genuinely love her. The irony of Holly Golightly's name notwithstanding, to this day, something in me cracks every time I watch this movie or reread Truman Capote's original story. As a child barreling into adolescence, I completely identified with Holly.

So it was that in junior high, with visions of Audrey Hepburn and George Peppard staking out the five-and-ten and fleeing in stolen Halloween masks, I graduated to shoplifting. The open bins at Woolworth's served as an invitation to help myself to LifeSavers, Cover Girl lipstick, Magic Markers. I pocketed tortoiseshell barrettes, samples of Blue Grass perfume. But it was no fun alone. If I could get away with it, I told my two best friends, surely we all could. As long as we just took cheap junk, no one would even care. Our shoplifting expeditions thrilled my friends once, twice, maybe three times, but they soon began to worry the counter ladies were onto them. They felt guilty. Fine, I said. Be that way. I went back briefly to solo theft, but it now felt too shameful.

I earned straight A's, ran for student council, edited the school literary magazine. I tried be good and fit in, yet felt this undertow of need to be bad and rebel. I longed for order and consistency, for rules that didn't contradict each other, and that I could trust as my own, but only one rule never seemed to vary:

If I stopped eating, I'd become thin. I'd no longer be that chubby child who looked and felt so out of control. I'd become as perfectly untouchable as Holly Golightly.

The role of sexual abuse as a catalyst for anorexia and bulimia nervosa has been searingly debated among eating disorders experts. According to Kelly Brownell, who directs the Yale Center for Eating and Weight Disorders, "There was a time when many people felt there was a one-to-one relationship, and that if anorexics said they hadn't been abused, it was because they'd repressed it. This was completely contrary to the science, but they were so devoted to this notion, you'd have shouting matches at professional meetings." What the research does show is that abuse of any kind puts a person at risk for lots of problems, bulimia nervosa—and to a much lesser extent anorexia—among them. Between 1989 and 1993, the National Institute on Drug Abuse surveyed more than three thousand women and found that more than half of those who were bulimic had been either raped, molested, or physically assaulted—compared to less than a third of those who had been anorexic or had no eating disorders. A 2004 Harvard study found that women with a history of childhood physical and sexual abuse were four times as likely to develop bulimia and binge eating disorders as other women. But Brownell warned against viewing any eating disorder as "proof" of abuse. "One's reaction to abuse depends not only on your particular temperament but the way your body and mind react to certain stresses." Many people who've been traumatized, he pointed out, use alcohol to numb themselves. "For them the chemical effect is reinforcing, but people who don't get that effect don't abuse alcohol. Dieting might be the same thing—restriction and control and perfectionism all have a different reinforcing mechanism for some people than for others."

By most reports, more than one fifth of *all* American women have some history of childhood sexual abuse. Girls with compulsive or impulsive temperaments may be more likely than others to turn to eating disorders as a coping strategy. They may be less likely to report the incident, especially if warned not to, and they may be more likely to blame and subconsciously punish themselves for what happened. Among the women I interviewed, however, sexual abuse was the exception rather than the rule. Yvonne Anderson, the comparative religion professor, told me that in her group-therapy sessions she'd actually felt twinges of envy for the women who'd been molested, because they had a concrete and understandable reason for their depression and eating disorders. They'd "earned" their shame, while she had no "right" to hers. Others, like the reclusive Kim Olensky, had only a vague—even amused—recollection of "experimentation" that occurred at a very young age. When Kim was four, her thirteen-year-old brother took her out in the yard and removed her clothes, but before he could get any further, they both were stung by hornets. Overall, the majority of people with histories of anorexia and bulimia have *no* history of abuse.

Shame, on the other hand, pervades eating disorders. According to British researchers Nicholas Troop and Lucy Serpell, both physical shame (*I need to hide my loathsome body*) and generalized shame (*I need to hide my loathsome thoughts*) play central roles in both anorexia and bulimia nervosa. Levels of self-loathing are most intense in those with active disorders; but as with anxiety, shame remains high even following the return to healthy eating. Because abuse is such an obvious cause of humiliation, some therapists jumped to conclusions. But self-loathing is both too variable and too common to signify any single cause. "Contained in the experience of shame," Gershen Kaufman writes in *Shame: The Power of Caring*, "is the piercing awareness of ourselves as fundamentally deficient in some vital way as a human being." It is this individual perception, rather than the specific act which prompts it, that is intrinsic to the psychology of eating disorders.

When I phoned my college classmate Gina Reed to ask what she thought lay at the root of her anorexia, her response was immediate and intense: "My family was a horror show." She told me her mother, the daughter of a rural Ohio farmer who believed in weekly canings, was a "rageaholic"who had been anorexic herself. In fact, she had dropped to 88 pounds at age nineteen—exactly the same weight Gina hit at that age. As a grown-up Mrs. Reed liked order and quiet, which did not come easy with three young children. Gina described the atmosphere in her family as "a constant state of disapproval" expressed through fits of fury . . . and long, icy silences.

No outsider could have guessed what was going on inside the Reed household, Gina said. Her mother didn't drink. Her father, a corporate lawyer, was rarely home. The family attended an Episcopal church every Sunday. Gina sang in the choir, and her brothers were altar boys. Her mother was their Scout leader, and all three children made the honor roll. The favorite of the family was the eldest son, Doug, a skinny, freckled boy with luminous green eyes. "When Mom went into a rage, it was Ned she beat. Doug only got hit when she felt compelled to punish all her children equally."

Each evening, like most housewives in the suburbs of Boston, Gina's mother drove to the train station to pick up her commuter husband. Sometimes it took an hour for her to bring him home. During this time she left Doug in charge of Ned and Gina. One night when Gina was seven and Ned ten, Doug told them to come with him down to the unfinished basement.

"Lie down," he ordered his sister, "on your back."

She objected. The cold and damp came right through her cotton dress from the cement floor. The room smelled dead. Her braids felt like hard ropes under her shoulders, and the light from the naked overhead bulb burned her eyes.

Doug laughed. "Just do it. Ned, you lie down on top of her. . . . You'll see. It's fun."

It wasn't, but Gina went along because Doug was eleven and her mother had left him in charge. And because he said she was supposed to like it and there was something wrong with her if she didn't. And Ned didn't object, even though Doug made him do it.

Gina went along *for the next four years* as Doug watched or exposed himself while directing Ned to touch her. She went along because she didn't know any rules that allowed her to say no. One evening the door swung open, and their mother stood blinking down as her younger son bolted back from her naked daughter. Inexplicably, this did not send Mrs. Reed into one of her rages. She simply closed the door.

No one in the family ever directly acknowledged the molestation. The word *therapy* was never uttered. All that changed was that Gina now had to go along with her mother to the station. "It felt as if I was the one being punished."

By the time she entered junior high, Gina was able to avoid her brothers. She pulled into her schoolwork and otherwise kept quiet. In her junior year—the first year both brothers were away at college—she developed a crush on one of the tough guys in school. He got a kick out of turning this little good girl on to drugs and alcohol. Her grades dropped accordingly, but she didn't care. The boyfriend broke up with her while driving her home from school the day before spring break. It was March, in Massachusetts. Snow still crusted the ground. But Gina wasn't trusted with a key to the house, so she had to wait in the cold for her mother to come home. Hours later, when Gina told her what had happened, her mother merely shrugged. Gina spent the entire vacation in her room. Maybe her mother knew best, she decided. She should have known better than to trust a boy. Any boy.

Over the next months, Gina brought her grades up. She withdrew from her friends. She ate only at dinner and stayed up late, writing and composing songs. At a music arts program that summer she earned the highest awards of recognition. By the fall of senior year Gina weighed 82 pounds.

"No one said a thing about my weight," she told me incredulously. When her periods had stopped, she actually tried to alert

her mother. "She was doing laundry. I said, 'I'm not having periods anymore,' and she started yelling at me—'You don't eat
enough! Goddammit, how come everything's going wrong in this
family?' Remember, though I didn't know it at the time, this is a
woman who herself stopped eating at precisely the same age."

She scheduled Gina for her first gynecological exam but
failed to give her any idea what to expect. The doctor was elderly, male, and indifferent. He ordered her to put her feet in the
stirrups, spread her legs, and stare at the "birdies" floating in
the mobile above her head. "There I was again on my back on
the basement floor." Gina's voice shook over the phone as she
recalled the flashback thirty years earlier. "Again, I felt as if my
mother was punishing me."

She wanted to disappear. Bingeing and purging would have
been too gratifying. "It was all about abstinence and shame."

As soon as Gina graduated, her father accepted a job transfer abroad. Her parents sold the family home and packed for Europe. On their way to the airport, the Reeds dropped their
daughter at Yale to begin her freshman year. They gave her the
name of a local gynecologist, with instructions to check in with
him regularly.

The doctor was another elderly stranger, and Gina braced for
another round of humiliation. But this man didn't make her
take off her clothes. He asked her instead into his office. The
room smelled of cherry pipe tobacco and was full of books and
dark wood furniture, pictures of the doctor's family on the walls,
and a diploma from a school she didn't recognize. He asked
what she was studying. Did she miss her parents? Was she making friends?

"He talked to me." Even now a note of wonder crept into
Gina's voice as she remembered this gentle man. Each week for
an hour she would come by and sit across the desk from him.
"He asked me what I was reading. I still remember that. It
seemed so . . . kind."

Gina began to eat. But even as her weight crept up to 120

pounds, her shame burrowed deeper, waiting to emerge in new and more annihilating forms.

In graduate school Gina began dating the son of a four-star general, class valedictorian at the University of Michigan. "He won all-around everything and looked like Robert Redford. I thought I'd won the proverbial Big Man on Campus." But in retrospect Gina realizes that she should have known to stay away from Steve. Tall, slender, and green eyed, he looked like her brother Doug. To paraphrase Fairbairn, she was about to become a sinner in a world ruled by the Devil.

Gina hesitated, then put down the phone to make sure her two young children weren't home from school yet. Her voice hardened as she came back on. "One night we were out drinking with friends, and he entered me in a wet T-shirt contest at this bar up near the university. With enough beers he was able to persuade me it was just for fun."

It was such fun for him that he took her to a strip club next. "I convinced myself it was a curiosity tour. Steve insisted I get up and dance. I focused on the other women." There was a philosophy student from Grosse Pointe. A Salvadoran girl who refused to take off her crucifix. An unwed Nigerian mother of twins. "I interviewed them as if I were Gloria Steinem undercover. And when I got up onstage I just sort of tuned out."

I knew the feeling. Psychologists call it dissociation.

"Aimee"—her voice cracked—"we became regulars. Twice, three times a *week*."

"Why did you stay with him?"

"I told myself I was studying him, too. He was so bright politically, but intellectually as deep as the sidewalk. I couldn't figure him out. And that family. They had this gorgeous property by a river down in North Carolina, where everybody would gather for annual reunions. I went fishing with his aunt and grandmother for trout before breakfast. In the evenings his uncles sat around telling stories and singing. The kids—including Steve and me—all slept on the screened-in porch, guys at one end, girls at the other. I loved that place, those people. But the last night there, when I'd made up my mind to leave him, I felt as if I were developing a picture in a darkroom, watching a monster emerge."

"What finally made the difference?"

"He'd started bragging about me—the way Arnold Schwarzenegger would, you know? I convinced myself nobody knew, but then he took out an ad." The phone fell silent. She whispered, "He was advertising for men to come have sex with me in our apartment while he watched."

I pictured the slight, unassuming classics major I had known in college. "Oh, Gina . . . I am so, so sorry."

Several seconds passed in silence. "The thing is," she said finally, "I knew about that ad, and I still couldn't break away. People responded—you can imagine. Steve arranged to meet one of the men at this bar downtown. We walk in and I see a guy I know there. I try to hide, but he saw us. He saw the man we were meeting. I just looked at my friend's face and knew he *knew*. I told Steve no. It was over."

A few weeks later Gina began talk therapy. A decade after her anorexia, she had finally begun the long, uncertain process of reclaiming her life. That process, she readily admitted, was ongoing. "But fortunately, there is this part of me that no one ever touched. This happy part. It's like if you garden and you find this little seedling you'd forgotten about." I pictured Hannah's seed of sorrow. "You brush away the soil and put some light on it and you keep watering it, and it keeps growing. It didn't get messed around with because you kept it well hidden. Now you can take it out and let it grow. You'll be a late bloomer is all!" She laughed, but sobered quickly. "I'm luckier than my brothers."

A "league of pain," Gina called her family. It wasn't just the sexual abuse. It wasn't just the eating disorders. It wasn't only her mother's icy rages or her father's detachment. "With Doug it was constant torment." He finished college, married a dutiful wife, but he couldn't stop watching, exposing himself, especially to children. He rented a duplex owned by a family with pubescent daughters. He took them to the attic and took off their clothes. Both became anorexic, which prompted their parents to get them into treatment, which in turn exposed Doug's molestations. After he was reported to the police, his wife left him. He lost his job. His compulsive behaviors, of which hand washing has since become the most constant and obvious, escalated. Never prosecuted due to the statute of limitations, he went on medication, which he sometimes refuses to take. Through it all, his parents have supported him.

"Ned behaved more overtly. He did drugs. He was an alcoholic. He couldn't keep a job. He was arrested for stealing. He dropped out of three colleges. Finally, at fifty, he meets Mary Alice and they go off to Poughkeepsie, and he sells RVs and he's very happy living in this middle-middle-class subdivision. Her parents are close by. He likes her parents a lot. They're normal. They fight, they get over it.

"So much of the problem," Gina said, "comes from not being able to admit unhappiness, or to see that unhappiness is normal, to see that dissatisfaction and anger are normal. In my family there was only a small spectrum of emotion that was ever allowed to become public. Real, full emotions had to remain hidden. So if you're not allowed to tell the truth, you start thinking up internal kinds of solutions."

Mixed messages like the ones that echoed through generations of the Reed family today permeate our culture. The Catholic church exalts spiritual perfection while protecting pedophile priests. A nation that espouses "moral values" supports the world's largest pornography industry. But the doublespeak is hardly limited to sexuality. Children are protected by their parents far longer than they were a century ago, yet from preschool are pressured to compete in school, in sports, in contests to a degree that was unthinkable even in the 1970s. There are more opportunities for girls than ever, yet, as journalist Peggy Orenstein has documented, girls "receive the conflicting messages of silence and assertiveness at home, at school, from boys." Then, after they grow up, women are encouraged to lead companies, raise families, run marathons, meanwhile taking their fashion and fitness cues from models half their age—most of whom have been surgically enhanced or whose photos are air brushed. Too many of us are trained to be meek and taught to be daring, and the contradictions only intensify with social class and status.

The result is that we lose our center, even in the way we think. If we're not thin, we're fat. If we're not winners, we're losers. If we're not good, we must be evil—and the same goes for everyone around us. Psychologists call this "black-and-white thinking," and they warn that those who buy into this schema set themselves up for shame. No one buys in more wholeheartedly than people in the grip of anorexia and bulimia. As Marya Hornbacher writes: "It's hard to describe how these two things can take place in the same mind, the arrogant, self-absorbed pride in yourself for your incredible feat, and the belief that you are so evil as to deserve starvation and any other form of self-mutilation. They coexist because you've split yourself in two. . . . This is not psychosis, this splitting. It is the history of Western culture made manifest."

Freud coined the term *reaction formation* to describe some individuals' tendency to suppress urges by doing or saying exactly the opposite of their impulse. The anorexic's insistence that she is "not hungry" is a reaction formation, as is the sex addict's campaign against pornography or the alcoholic's righteous rage at the sight of his son drinking. Reaction formations are the internal corsets we tighten around unacceptable appetites—appetites that our culture, family, or superego persuades us should be an absolute zero. The problem is that appetites don't zero out. They exist for a reason. To perpetuate the species. To sustain life. To fuel civilization. Attempts to suppress them only create, in feminist Susan Bordo's words, "a war that tears the subject in two—a war explicitly thematized, by many anorexics, as a battle between the male and female sides of the self."

Yale psychologist Kelly Brownell once asked me how I had recovered from anorexia. I told him about my turning-point summer in New Haven, how, like most of my interviewees, I'd consciously chosen normalcy and retrained myself by watching what people I admired ate, how they talked and behaved—and sometimes misbehaved. I told him about one particular incident that occurred when I was twenty-two, a period when I was sexually promiscuous, still occasionally bulimic, and often felt the way Gina described: as if I were on a curiosity tour of someone else's life. This particular night a man I was dating had taken me along with some friends to a medieval theme restaurant. We sat at long wooden tables, filling our goblets with wine, as the waiter explained the rules. We could eat with our hands and yell for the "serving wenches," get up and dance and be rowdy as we liked. The waiter made a point of saying the one thing we were not to do was throw food. With that, as if issuing an invitation, he slid a long bread loaf down the center of the table. I promptly pulled off a foot length of bread and hurled it across the room.

Brownell studied me as if to visualize this bad girl. "How did that feel?"

"Exhilarating. Daring." I laughed. "Wicked. I will never forget the horror on my button-downed date's face. But the thrill only lasted a second, and then I was hideously ashamed." In fact, I drank my way silently through the rest of that dinner and afterward spent most of the night sitting in an empty bathtub, trying to sort out my confusion in my journal while my lover slept.

Dr. Brownell smiled. "Sometimes it's good to learn how to be a little bad. It's called getting real."

Part Two

THE PHYSICS
OF NORMALCY

Personal Relationship

6

A CERTAIN SELF
Identity and Independence

> The real struggle . . . is about *you*: you, a person who has to learn to live in the real world, to inhabit her own skin, to know her own heart, to stop waiting for her life to begin.
> —Caroline Knapp, *Appetites*

IT'S NOT EASY TO PIN BETSY KELLY DOWN. She spends months at a time on location in Thailand, South Africa, Peru, and Costa Rica. When back in LA she's usually either in the editing room or on the phone with her sponsors. She and her husband, Bill, produce documentaries about the environment and human rights. Work is a full-time affair. But when she learned I was writing this book, she took time out to have lunch with me at the café downstairs from her Beverly Hills production offices. She wanted to tell me her story, she said, because it was so unusual.

Though we didn't know each other as kids, Betsy and I share a number of common denominators. We both grew up in the suburbs of New York City and both now live in Los Angeles. We both married in our early twenties, both to older men—Bill is twenty years older than Betsy. Neither of us had been away from home for more than a weekend before we went to college. Neither of us drank, used drugs, or had sex in high school. But my history of anorexia more closely matched that of Betsy's younger sister Anne, who began aggressively dieting at thirteen. Betsy didn't start obsessing about weight until college, at which point Anne, with the confounding defensiveness that so often prompts girls to cling to anorexia as an identity, told her, "This is mine. You can't have it."

Betsy assured her sister she didn't want her problem. Unlike Anne and me, Betsy hated being too thin. Once the compulsion to lose weight began, however, she couldn't stop. While Anne and I both quit our eating disorders without treatment as we entered our twenties, Betsy sought professional help and spent four years in therapy.

Now forty, Betsy looks thirty. Her hair falls in auburn waves to her shoulders. Freckles dust her cheeks. A small gold cross hangs at her throat, and the day we met she wore a plaid shirt-dress, not too tight and not too loose, not too formal and not too casual, and neither overtly sexy nor chic. The dress's style and bright autumnal colors stood out among the clipped black outfits of our fellow diners, mostly talent agents and movie industry executives, who were picking over their endive and arugula salads. I suspect we were not the only ones with histories of eating disorders in this power-lunch setting.

I asked Betsy to take me back to the beginning. "What did you think when Anne got sick?"

"I didn't get it." As a teenager Betsy had no illusions about her size or maturity. "I was thin, but I was never going to be like my mother or sister heightwise or bodywise. I always considered myself the bigger one in the family."

I reminded her she wasn't exactly a stranger to obsessiveness. She'd told me she used to wash her hands incessantly as a teenager.

"Mm . . . and I did have a little tendency to count things. I had to have a certain number of things. When I was about ten, if I got nervous, I'd twitch one eye."

"Twitch one eye?"

She shrugged. "It made me feel better. The weird thing is that I never made the connection at the time, that I was doing it *in order* to feel better."

As Betsy talked about her family, more connections emerged. The Kellys lived clean. They kept no pets. Kissing on the lips was not allowed. If anybody got a cold when the kids were little, everybody had to wear surgical masks—Betsy's dad was a public health doctor. In the basement, out of view from visitors, Betsy's mother meticulously saved and organized old *Life* and *Time* magazines, rubber bands, broken china, shoes, the children's elementary school homework, as well as scraps of paper. She kept the house cold to conserve fuel, and made curtains and most of her clothes but used only the most expensive fabrics, which she bought at discount. At mass on Sunday, the family looked as if they'd just stepped off the cover of *Town & Country*. "We lived above our means. The message to us kids was, we could do whatever we wanted for a living as long as we made over a hundred thousand dollars." When Betsy was twenty she casually asked her internist if her height and weight were normal. He said, "Yes, but if you wanted to work out or run a little . . ." Betsy overreacted.

"I wanted to lose five pounds," she explained. "Before I knew it I was using diuretics, compulsively exercising, and aggressively dieting. I never experienced the temptation to be bulimic, and I never got under one hundred pounds, but I couldn't stop the obsessiveness. If I didn't get a certain amount of exercise or didn't count every calorie I was eating, it was so upsetting that it was just easier to do it. It made me crazy. Still, I never realized how broad the compulsion was until I went to the doctor, and he asked if I had other obsessions."

By then she'd been trapped in the syndrome for four years and was three years into marriage, which had intensified her compulsions along with her stress level. Not only was her husband twice her age, but he had two children, one almost as old as she was. Their mother, an alcoholic, tried to turn them against Betsy. Her own parents didn't hide their disapproval. Shortly after the wedding, she and Bill moved across country. Because Bill at the time was a concert promoter, Betsy was expected suddenly to socialize as a professional wife. Self-conscious about her age, she tried to seem more sophisticated and stronger than she really was. Simultaneously, she could not stop thinking about how she had to shrink her body.

Her love for her husband, Betsy emphasized, was never in doubt. But it helped that he played an active role in her therapy. "Bill had gone through the addiction of his first wife, so he understood how important treatment was. He came to my therapy sessions and went through therapy himself. We talked about everything, which helped our marriage immensely when I came out of it."

Betsy was treated at the UCLA Eating Disorders Program. Even under the care of experts, however, recovery from her disorder was not quick. Therapy helped Betsy and her husband explore their expectations of each other. She renegotiated her relationship with her stepchildren, reminding herself that their resistance didn't necessarily mean she was bad or had done anything wrong. She learned how to defend herself against their mother's criticism. Still, the obsessive thoughts about dieting and exercise kept drumming inside her head. Finally, after about two years of talk therapy, her doctor suggested she try Prozac. Her weight at that point was 105, giving her enough body mass on her five-foot-seven frame to respond well to medication. Research on Prozac suggested it could reduce her obsessional thinking and help prevent relapses of anorexia later on.

Betsy resisted her doctor's advice. "I was raised to believe you better be dying even to take an aspirin. I didn't like the idea that I'd be dependent on a drug and have to give up control. I'm generally stubborn about control."

Hard to find an anorexic who isn't, I pointed out.

But eventually she agreed to try medication. "Once I made the leap of faith to go ahead and start it, I immediately felt stronger. That gave me the ability not to quit." This determination was important, since the chemical benefits took about four weeks to kick in, and there were some initial side effects while the dosage was being adjusted. "I did get very sleepy at first. I also had incredibly vivid dreams, and occasionally my heart raced as if I were having a panic attack. In the morning when I first took the pills my voice seemed louder to me and my speech sounded a bit frenetic." Also in the beginning, Prozac affected Betsy's libido. "It was more difficult to orgasm. It wasn't impossible—it just took longer." None of these side effects lasted more than a few months, however.

Meanwhile, the drug arrested not only Betsy's obsession with dieting but also her other compulsions—hand washing, checking herself in the mirror, counting, and making lists of minutiae. As Betsy's obsessions faded, her self-confidence rose.

It sounded like a miracle cure. "So was that the end of therapy?"

"More like a fresh start. Prozac helped me gain back enough control to deal with issues with a clearer head." The paradox, of course, is that Betsy's lack of control had been caused by her obsession with control.

Her therapist had Betsy write out her life, much as I had done in *Solitaire*. "Every detail—as I remembered it—from day one." In the process, she realized she was as much of a perfectionist as her sister and her mother, and that her parents' subtle but steady pressure promoted this compulsion. "My mother would praise me for doing well in school. I never really enjoyed school, so I'd say, 'I did well because I had to do well.' She'd say, 'No. You did well because you wanted to do well.' I'd say, 'No. No, I really didn't.' I never said it, but what I was thinking was, *Don't tell me what I want!*" Betsy graduated from high school in three years, and her father immediately began planning for her to do the same in college so she could start med school before she was twenty. By the time it dawned on her she didn't actually want to be a doctor she was anorexic.

As she wrote out her history, Betsy felt free for the first time to tell the whole truth of her life as she saw it. She also gained new insights into her sister. Although Anne had quit anorexia at twenty, claiming she "just got sick of it," she continued to exercise compulsively. She resisted intimacy and so tended to cycle through relationships. Betsy tried to tell her what she'd discovered in therapy, but Anne refused to consider treatment. "Only now in her mid-thirties," Betsy told me, "after another bad breakup, is she finally seeing a therapist and beginning to deal with the reasons why her life is in pieces."

"Well, if you had to advise her," I said, "which part of your treatment was the most important? Prozac or writing out your life story?"

Betsy leaned forward. "I would honestly suggest to *everyone* that writing down your own account of your life is an invaluable experience. It allows you to reconnect with yourself and examine what's actually happened to you, and finally to let yourself feel things in reexperiencing them."

"So tell me why you're still on Prozac."

"One example. If nine people say something positive and one says something negative, it's the negative I hear. No question. Prozac doesn't stop that, but it takes the emotional edge off." If she goes off it, that hypersensitivity returns. "I did try," Betsy said. "After about four years I tried to lower the dosage from forty milligrams—but I noticed a return of hand-washing desire, the sensitivity, and circular thinking—so I've stayed at forty milligrams."

She thought for a minute and then said, "Perhaps what helped me most, what allowed me to persist until I found the right combination of treatments, was that I never lost sight of the goal of wanting to get back to normal."

*   *   *

The thirst for normalcy is often a first signal of recovery. What triggers this thirst, however, can be as variable as human experience. Greer Wallace recalled her grandmother driving her back to college after Greer had spent the summer refusing to eat. Her grandmother casually invited her to share a milkshake when they stopped for a break in the two-day journey, and the offer was made with such unconditional love that Greer was overwhelmed by nostalgia for her childhood. Back then, when she felt normal, she would have leaped at her grandmother's offer without a second thought. The memory cracked the shell of her anorexia, and she ate a little to please her grandmother. A week or two later, an introductory class in architecture provided an even more powerful incentive. Architecture spoke to Greer's penchant for order and precision but also aroused her love of beauty and design. If she became an architect, she sensed, she could be herself, authentic and engaged, and also feel normal as an adult in the world. Suddenly, she had—in effect—something to eat for. Much as Lucy Romanello, the Chicago divinity graduate, had chosen her husband and religious faith over anorexia, Greer chose normalcy in the form of a career she adored. She went on to build her own firm and over nearly thirty years has never doubted the rightness of her choice.

I remember that when I began to recover, normalcy beckoned like a klieg light marking a Hollywood wrap party. I could make it out in the distance and knew that others were enjoying the celebration, but a darkened city without signposts separated me from the festivity. The only way to the light was through the darkness, and that meant taking risks. I chose to follow the example of Holly Golightly.

"Traveling," Holly's calling card had read, and in my first four years after college I aspired to the same. I moved three times in Manhattan, worked for a stock analyst, quit painting, took up writing, waited tables from Beekman Place to SoHo. I moved to Chicago, worked as a flight attendant for three years, and published my first book, then began writing for business magazines. By the time I was twenty-eight, my travels had landed me in Los Angeles with my future husband.

That winter, returning to Boston to visit my college roommate Patty, I felt downright full of myself. I had succeeded, or so it seemed, in becoming a woman of poise and worldliness. In fact, I had moved into grown-up normalcy faster even than Patty, without whom I'd probably still have been wandering hungrily around the Yale campus. It was Patty, consummate procrastinator that she was, who taught me it was possible to graduate from Yale with honors without obsessing over exams and that ambition and pleasure did not have to be mutually exclusive. After college Patty became a public defender. But into her late twenties she had also maintained the social life of a student. Now, when she brought me to a party of her fellow lawyers in Cambridge, I felt as if I were sliding seven years into the past. This had an unsettling effect on me.

The party was held in a one-bedroom walk-up with Aerosmith blasting, smoke swirling, and couples sipping from plastic cups, pretending they could hear each other. Dope was being puffed on the fire escape, cocaine sniffed in the bathroom. All but married, with a soon-to-be stepson in preschool, I'd almost forgotten how much voltage a crowd of single men and women could generate. I was relieved when, after an hour or so, Patty asked if I wanted to leave. But then she struck up a conversation with a young law clerk. As she was introducing me, my gaze strayed past her into the kitchen. I spotted a face I recognized.

Mortified, I excused myself, said I'd meet Patty outside, and withdrew to fetch my coat. Ben—the man in the kitchen—had been a casual acquaintance in college, a classmate with a crooked smile and fuzzy hair who occasionally sat at my table in the dining hall. Once or twice I danced with him at mixers, and it felt awkward because he was a full head shorter than I. None of that, however, was what now sent me racing for the door. Logically, in fact, I should have pressed in the opposite direction to hail him as an old friend. But I was too ashamed. Still shorter than me, Ben was—I feared—several pounds lighter than my current weight of 128. I imagined myself through his eyes: gargantuan. I could not bear it.

So I thought at the time. Looking back on this peculiar reaction more than twenty years later, I realize it had little to do with Ben. It had a great deal, however, to do with another Yale man I'd dated six years earlier. Allen and I had met when I was twenty-three and still living in New York. He said he used to see me when we were both in college, and though he'd never talked to me then, he liked what he saw. The girl he remembered weighed 100 pounds. When our affair began I weighed 120. Allen was then finishing his residency in plastic surgery. Our final day together he flipped open a *Mademoiselle* magazine, pointed to a model in a Chanel ad, and asked me, "How much weight do you think you'd have to lose to look like that?"

Today I can speculate that the question might, in his mind, have been clinical. This, after all, was a man who used silicone breast implants for paperweights. He kept that *Mademoiselle* and the stacks of *Vogue* and *Harper's Bazaar* underneath it as reference materials. Allen was going into the business of repackaging human beings. He would make a handsome living "transforming" normal women into imitations of the models in those magazines, and he actually believed this to be a noble occupation. So it is conceivable that his arrogance and insensitivity were unwitting, but as far as I was concerned they were also unforgivable. Regrettably, my anger played second to my humiliation, and now in Boston the heat of that insult branded me all over again. Even though I knew better, I couldn't bear for another man from my past to see what had become of the "perfection" that used to be me.

"I'm too old for this," I told Patty when she found me.

"For what?" She followed my gaze back through the door to Ben, who still had not noticed us.

"He won't recognize me."

"What are you talking about?" Compact, soft-armed, with a

dimpled chin and wide brown eyes, Patty looked and probably weighed the same as she had the day she graduated.

"He knew me as this little . . . *wisp*."

"And good for you—you've grown out of it. Go say hello!"

I stared in at the wall of strangers. Ben had moved out of sight. "I can't," I said.

Eating disorders sabotage identity. This, in turn, can sabotage recovery, as therapists frequently find when treating patients with medication alone. Although antidepressants can be very effective in stopping bingeing and purging, many bulimics will quit their medication after only a few weeks, in order to "get back" their eating disorder. "To these patients," Steven Levenkron writes in *Anatomy of Anorexia*, "their disease had become part of their life, their identity, and assisted them in creating a sense of emotional balance. Rationally, they wanted to get rid of the disease; but emotionally, they missed it, as if they had lost a close friend."

"This is the pitiful stage where you do not qualify as an eating-disordered person," Marya Hornbacher recalls. "And you feel bad about this. You feel as if you really *ought* to count, you ought to still merit worry." Caroline Knapp called it "the post-anorexic riddle of identity, a sense of wild shapelessness."

Health, according to anorexic logic, equals a loss of status, of specialness, but perhaps most important, of clarity. You've failed to exert the ultimate willpower, failed to pare your body and soul down to its true essence, failed to sustain that incandescent identity as a creature who defies definition—not to mention the very laws of nature. You've failed to reduce yourself to a perfect object. The knowledge that this identity was impossible, demeaning, and false offers scant consolation, for it still leaves the gaping question, Who *are* you? For years you'll move along just fine, gaining weight, gaining confidence, gaining all the trappings of a thriving life, and then, unexpectedly, a shadow of your past will resurface in the face of a long-lost friend or a moment of revived anxiety, and your bright new self will cringe, yearning for that old mask of "perfection."

To fully recover from an eating disorder, Sheila Reindl wrote in *Sensing the Self*, "a woman has to lose her conception of who she thought she was or thought she should be. . . . She has to relinquish her effort to craft a constructed self and instead must let herself be who she is." Reindl based this observation on more than twenty years of experience, as a counselor at Harvard University's campus counseling center and as a clinical psychologist and researcher. Since her study was one of the few I found to focus on life *after* bulimia, I wanted to ask her why she thought this question of identity was so often so fraught.

Reindl suggested we meet at her office in Cambridge. Unlike the bureaucratic university cubicles where I typically interviewed researchers, the room's soft lighting, combined with Reindl's contemplative demeanor, nudged me to think like a patient. Before I quite realized it, I was telling her about that 1981 party with Patty, which had taken place just blocks from where we now sat. "It was almost like a panic attack," I recalled, "this explosion of shame at the prospect of facing someone who had last seen me at a hundred pounds. The thing was, I couldn't tell whether I was more ashamed for having been anorexic or for having recovered."

Reindl studied me before she answered. "Recovery is like a big old house," she said finally. "The anorexic or the bulimic is always going to live there. People sometimes think, I can evict her, I can get rid of that. But you don't develop an eating disorder for no good reason. It's a profound experience. So how could you wipe out that whole piece of your history? I prefer to think of it this way. She used to rule the house in a kind of tyranny. She was in charge of the kitchen, in charge of everything. Now she still gets to live there and she may still have some of those old fears and vulnerabilities, but she's got only one room in the house and has to make way for more and more occupants as time passes."

Reindl's use of metaphor intrigued me. In *Sensing the Self* she'd spent an entire chapter drawing parallels between the experience of bulimics and the fairy tale "Beauty and the Beast." To reach a happy ending, she argued, both in the fairy tale and in bulimia, the Beast of natural appetite, impulse, and ugliness has to be acknowledged and "wedded" to the more socially acceptable Beauty of good behavior, social restraint, and idealized looks.

"We all have to integrate the light with the dark," Reindl said, "the noble and ignoble aspects of ourselves. That's a normal developmental task. It's just harder for people with eating disorders." With anorexia, the act of losing weight serves as a metaphor for the feeling that one is emotionally invisible. "The kid who's going to become anorexic typically takes pride in her disciplined emptiness, imagining it as perfect beauty. So the message for her is that you don't have to be perfect to be loved. The bulimic, on the other hand, binges and purges in secret—hiding the beast she knows is in there. The issues of shame are stronger. I think that's why, when anorexics hit a bulimic patch in recovery or difficulties even later in life, they often want to go back to the anorexia. It felt cleaner and tidier—they didn't have to deal with all these messy feelings and conflicts."

The most enduring obstacle to health in the aftermath of anorexia and bulimia, Reindl believes, is the question of *enough*. "The women in my study—one to four years after recovery—were still vulnerable to the sense of not being enough, not having enough, not knowing when enough is enough. It's confusing because you need to accept yourself as you are and yet keep striving to embrace more of who you are."

"That sounds like enough *means* more."

She smiled. "It also means separating feeling from judgment. I meet so many people who are afraid of feeling pain, of having their heart broken, of loneliness. They're afraid pain mirrors something bad in themselves. It must mean I'm unlovable, unworthy. Maybe it just means, I'm lonely."

* * *

Researchers often say that genetics load the "gun" of eating disorders, and environment "pulls the trigger." The stories of anorexia and bulimia I've heard, however, convince me that this metaphor needs a little tweaking. It seems to me that genetics *make* the gun, and the cultural and familial environment *loads* it, but it takes the experience of unbearable *emotion* to pull the trigger. Of these three elements, the experience of emotion most immediately determines our sense of normalcy. It is also the force over which we have the most control—hard though this may be for someone in the grip of an eating disorder to believe.

Loneliness, guilt, fear, and shame were as inextricable as they were inescapable in Megan Rainer's memory of anorexia. Today she dates that memory from the year she turned fourteen, the first year she ever went on a diet. But age fourteen was also the first year she remembers feeling depressed and, crucially, the first year she understood that she and her identical twin, Polly, were two different people. "I realized Polly was far more comfortable in her skin than I was."

"What made you think so?" I asked.

"I'd watch boys flirt with her."

There was an unmistakable note of sadness in Megan's voice. Even at fifty, it seemed, she equated how Polly felt *in* her skin with how men looked *at* Polly's body. I thought of Jean-Paul Sartre's analysis of perception: "Through the Other's look I *live* myself as fixed in the midst of the world." But as a twin, Megan seemed to take this a step farther. "Polly's always been more at ease with herself, but because I thought of us as one person—if she had that comfort level, I couldn't."

Megan's own experience with men seemed to confirm this split. "Freshman year of college I found my boyfriend in bed with another woman. Then I discovered that two guys I had dated in high school had been having sexual relationships with other people while they were with me. Meanwhile, I was still a virgin. I remember thinking, they don't like me that way. I wasn't mature enough to challenge them. Instead, I lost twenty pounds. If men were never going to look at me, then I would make it obvious why they shouldn't. I didn't have a single date after freshman year. Anorexia was all about rejection. And separation. And control."

I thought of Jen's comment thirty years earlier on the lawn of Science Hill: First, admit what you want. "Why control," I asked Megan, "but not power?"

"Oh, I think that's huge!" She paused. Megan today is a staunch feminist and women's advocate. Yet she admitted, "Power scares the shit out of me. Being a powerful woman scares me. Being controlled is disarming—diminutive and weak and safe. There's a Cinderella syndrome at work. You know, *If they only knew? I'm fooling everybody*. That's the opposite of power. It undermines one's power."

"So what made you finally realize that?"

"Well, my first big wake-up call was my husband Carl. Once he started calling me by the right name, that is." She laughed. Carl's first word to her was "Polly?" The occasion was Polly's engagement party, and Carl was a friend of her fiancé. "It was not an easy night for me anyway," Megan recalled. "That made me so furious, I just stormed away." Carl tried to make it up by taking Megan dancing. A few days later he challenged her to tennis. They went camping and argued about the Greeks and the galaxies and Thomas Merton. Suddenly, at twenty-eight, Megan felt deeply connected to someone who wasn't her sister or her parent. Carl helped her to see herself from a whole new vantage point. She felt authentic. She felt real and whole.

That view acquired ever more dimension as Megan began to see herself through the eyes of colleagues and students at the community college where she teaches art history, and, eventually, through her two children. But even today, the old gap in perception can still open up, especially around the issue of sexuality. "I wore a dress just a couple of nights ago, much more revealing than most of my clothes, and my daughter goes, 'Mom, that's great. You look so sexy!' But, you know, I had to squelch the impulse to go in and change. I want to feel sexy, and I do with my husband, but not otherwise."

She paused. "Even now a little thing like that will freak me out and I'll be tempted to sabotage everything I've gained."

In 2000 University of Michigan researchers Karen Stein and Linda Nyquist asked a group of twenty-six recovering anorexics, fifty-three bulimics, and thirty-four healthy women with no history of eating disorders to define themselves. Each woman was given a stack of fifty-two cards and asked to write a different description of herself on each one. Some possible examples: *good student, sexpot, picky eater, chubby teenager, strong runner, clumsy dancer.* Then she was asked to code each description as positive, negative, or neutral and rank its relative importance as a measure of how she saw herself. Women with histories of anorexia and bulimia were nearly four times as likely as other women to create a strongly negative self-portrait. But their self-negation went far beyond body dissatisfaction. The eating disordered saw themselves overall as less competent, less intelligent, less popular, and less happy human beings.

Such misgivings are by no means limited to women or to whites or to middle-class Americans—or to heterosexuals. "I remember approaching my mom when I was five," Chiao-min Lee told me. "I asked her, 'Do you ever feel like you don't belong somewhere?' I didn't mean in the community but physically in my body. Looking back, I think what I was feeling was depression. This empty feeling where sadness just begins to grow. I never felt my body matched my gender—who I was on the inside. I wanted a sex change operation before I was ten. I identified more with women, with dolls, the female form. I never saw myself growing up to be a man." But Chiao-min was growing up—in the mostly white conservative middle-class culture of Bakersfield, California. "I experienced a lot of racial taunts when I was younger. I was very small, very skinny. Very effeminate looking and acting." Finally, in high school he found a group of Asian students. But to become a member, to feel protected, to feel Asian American enough, he had to camouflage himself. The group was a gang. "Baggy clothing, this arrogant walk, this look. I went from trying to fit into a group of white kids to fitting in with this Asian group that was masculine, sexist, and violent. We never wielded guns, but we got into fights, talked about women as if they were crap. I knew I wasn't straight, but I hid the fact all through high school."

Chiao-min came out at nineteen, the beginning of what he calls his second adolescence. His mother's immediate response was, "Don't ever tell your father. He'll kill himself." Instead, she took control and told his dad, who then asked Chiao-min's straight brother how to react. Chiao-min's father assured him he loved him, but the two men haven't mentioned his sexuality in the ten years since. "I was never going to be good enough in my parents' eyes," Chiao-min told me, "but I kept thinking, What can I do to be better, to reach perfection in my own way?" He had always been thin and, when depressed as a child, tended to lose weight, but he only began actively trying to lose after coming out. "When you go to the clubs you see people with these bodies, and you think, Look how much attention they're getting. If they can accomplish that, why can't I? What's wrong with me?" He decided his body was wrong, restricted himself to one meal a day, and by twenty-two had a body fat ratio of 5 percent. The minimum standard for men, even if they are ultramarathoners, is 6.

What's wrong with me? If there were an anthem for eating disorders, this would be the chorus. What's wrong with me that I can't starve away? Or exercise away? Or stuff into silence? What's wrong with me that I can't feel, that I can't express— that I can't get rid of? The answer ultimately comes down to sensation. "I feel like an outsider in my own body" was how one woman put it. Psychiatrist Mark Warren elaborated: "It's as if visual sensation has overwhelmed all other sensation. There's a total distrust of smell, touch, taste, feel."

Warren's program at the Cleveland Center for Eating Disorders uses an approach called dialectical behavior therapy, or DBT, to bring eating disorder patients "back to the surface of sensation." Developed by Marsha Linehan in the early 1990s at the University of Washington, DBT was first designed for patients with borderline personality disorder. It combines techniques from Gestalt therapy, which focuses on the experience and acceptance of bodily sensation; behavioral therapy, which uses conditioning to change behavior, such as obsessive dieting; and cognitive therapy, which uses a systematic approach to change destructive beliefs, such as the idea that only thin people can be good, moral, or happy. Linehan accepted that self-defeating behaviors such as bingeing and purging, cutting, excessive exercise, or crash dieting are attempts to "solve" extreme emotional discomfort and that these behaviors do produce a biochemical sensation of relief for some people. They actually work up to a point, which is why they persist. "Just say no" is not a solution; therapy has to offer an alternative that works at least as well as the compulsion.

DBT works by training patients to trace the chain of events that lead up, say, to a binge, so they can figure out how and why their emotions unravel. A patient may have stayed up after midnight watching a movie; woken up too late to have breakfast; had too much coffee; and skipped lunch to study for a big test, which she did poorly on; and then come home so ravenous and frustrated that she binged and purged. In DBT, she'd connect these dots, then map out changes she might make to prevent the next binge: go to bed early, eat breakfast and lunch, reduce her caffeine intake, study ahead of time. As tediously commonsensical as this may sound, it can come as a revelation to people who have never stopped to consider their behavior and emotions as an interlocking puzzle (I'm thinking of almost any adolescent I've ever known). "Learn to be in control of your mind, instead of letting your mind control you" is a central tenet of DBT. To this end, therapists work with patients to recognize the difference between physical appetite and emotional appetite, between what they actually want and what they think they're supposed to want, and between what they can change and what is not only impossible but unnecessary to change.

The behavioral emphasis of DBT is on simple strategies such as eating controlled amounts of healthy foods at intervals throughout the day (a tactic that has been proven in study after study to prevent both undereating and overeating); practicing yoga, meditation, and mindfulness training to calm anxiety; and "distress tolerance" tactics, such as holding an ice cube instead of cutting or other forms of self-harm. The ultimate goal, Warren told me, is to equip the patient to experience sensation as a source of pleasure, comfort, and information, instead of as sheer anxiety.

With the same objective in mind, Harvard psychiatrist David Herzog recommends pets. "Touch is such a big issue," he explained. "Can I trust you to touch me? Can I trust myself to touch? But a pet knows no boundaries. What do you do when your dog licks your face? Experimenting is crucial. It's good to get a little dirty and smelly."

As he was talking I thought of the photograph of Caroline Knapp, who had been Herzog's patient, holding her dog, Lucille, on the flap of her memoir, *Pack of Two: The Intricate Bond Between People and Dogs*. "Put a leash in my hand," Knapp wrote some twenty years after her "anorexic phase," "put Lucille by my side, and something happens, something magical; something clicks inside, as though some key piece of me, missing for years, has suddenly slid into place, and I know I'll be okay." No wonder she thanked David Herzog in her acknowledgments.

"It's important to play with control," he told me, "to let yourself experience excess, to know you can bear it."

That same objective is behind the increasing use of horses in residential eating disorder programs. Equine therapy is predicated on the fact that horses are by nature "excessive" in size, yet as animals of prey they are also exquisitely sensitive to any fear, stress, or confusion in the humans who handle them. To calm a horse, the handler must herself become calm and focused. "She has to express herself," explained Carolyn Costin, who uses equine therapy with her clients at Monte Nido, an eating disorder treatment center. "She has to trust her own ability. And she cannot hide."

At Monte Nido, clients are assigned exercises in the ring—to persuade the horse to step over a board, for example, or go through a gateway—all without speaking. People with anorexia, Costin said, tend to come at these problems from the opposite direction than people with bulimia. "We had one client being treated for bulimia who was always in a hurry. She was impatient with other people, wanted to push ahead in therapy before she was ready." Staff members had tried to help this woman slow herself down, but she could not see that she was always racing. In the ring she was instructed to approach the horse and, using nonverbal commands, persuade the animal to back up. She moved so quickly and her body language was so erratic that the horse was stymied. "And the trainer, who's never met her in his life, says, 'You seem very impatient, as if it's hard for you to let things go at their own pace.' " The young woman resisted the trainer's message, but she couldn't argue with the horse. The only way she could complete the exercise was by slowing down and paying close attention to what she was thinking; how she was moving; and, most important, what she was feeling. People suffering from anorexia, by contrast, tend to be quiet and timid. Costin told me about one teenager whose exercise required her to signal the horse by waving her arms. "The girl lifted her hands a teeny bit, and the horse just stood there, like, I don't know what you're doing. So the trainer said gently, 'If you want to be understood you have to get the message across.' " Little by little the girl made herself more present until the horse began to respond.

One of the first programs to use equine therapy for eating

disorders was Remuda Ranch, in Wickenburg, Arizona. Each patient at Remuda is assigned to a particular horse and rides two to three times a week. Sharon Simpson, who directs Remuda's fifteen-year-old equine program, believes the bond that develops between horse and rider creates a sense of unconditional acceptance that many patients have never experienced before. Perfection has no place in this relationship. Metaphor, however, does. "The horse is a living, breathing animal," Simpson told me, "and because of that, he can be unpredictable, just like life is unpredictable."

Ruth Zimmerman, once bulimic, now, at twenty-five, has two horses of her own. Ruth believes that the power of equine therapy stems partly from the fact that the horse is neither independent nor subservient. "You have this one-on-one relationship with this creature who's never going to hurt you. It's never going to be competitive, and it's never going to be sexual or any of the threatening things that a human relationship can be." But it is emotionally intimate and, crucially, honest. "The slightest movement, the horse will feel. If you get tense or scared, even if you're just standing next to the horse, the horse gets scared. On the other hand, my horses will come over if they hurt me by accident. They know and they feel bad. It's a very reflective, symbiotic relationship."

"Exposure." That was Rob Martin's answer when I asked his greatest fear. Because he was a man, this surprised me. Because he'd been anorexic, perhaps it shouldn't have.

Rob and I met at a writers' conference where I was talking about this book. He said he knew someone I might like to interview. As we were leaving the room, he approached me and lowered his voice. "Of course, the person I want you to interview is me."

I had no idea. Rob was in his fifties, balding, of medium build; an articulate, engaging family doctor writing his first novel. And he was a straight male. Thanks to the myth that only gays suffer from body image problems, few heterosexual men will admit if they have an eating disorder. In fact, gays make up only about one fifth of all men with eating disorders, and men generally account for up to 15 percent of anorexia and bulimia nervosa cases. I knew that male jockeys, weight lifters, gymnasts, and runners frequently develop eating disorders as they struggle to "make weight." But Rob didn't fall into any of these categories. And that's precisely why he wanted to talk to me.

"I was never identified," he said, "never received one comment from one person, ever. Not on my obsessional eating, nothing. I look back on that in absolute amazement. It's an invisible problem among men."

In many ways, Rob's experience followed the classic contours of anorexia. "My mother has an eating disorder, never diagnosed, never acknowledged. 'I've been on a diet for sixty years' is how she would put it. She's five foot five and has weighed 105 her whole life. Her license plate says ENDURE. That's how she sees the world—be strong by resisting." She could also be described, he said, as an overprotective Jewish mother who wanted only the best for her son. Breaking away to college was hard. At seventeen, Rob became obsessed with weight loss and exercise. He'd eat nothing for a week but skinless chicken, then binge and drink heavily, then fast for days. Over two years he pared his five-foot-nine-inch body down to 117 pounds. Eventually, he began having trouble concentrating on his studies. His grades dropped enough to alarm him, and he forced himself to eat more regularly. But he didn't broaden his diet and he never sought therapy. Soon he was just as obsessive about maintaining as he had been about losing. Throughout college and into his first year of medical school he weighed all of 125 pounds. And he still had an abhorrence of fat that extended to being touched or seen naked. "Even now, I still can dislike my body. I know it's not true and I know it's wrong but I still have those feelings."

"So there you were in med school," I said, "shrinking from

your own body, yet you wanted to go into a profession that would force you to touch other people?"

He laughed. "Isn't that incredible? But I think a lot of doctors go into medicine because they're in denial about their own health issues. It's a way of trying to make yourself invulnerable."

Perfect for a man who's anorexic, I thought.

"It didn't work, though. Even after my weight stabilized, I had a profound awareness that something was bad about the way I organized the world." He took a leave from med school after his first year and worked with the undergraduate theater department at Rutgers. "They were putting on a production of *The Wizard of Oz*, and one day this freshman dancer showed up for rehearsal. She was wearing cutoffs and had bare feet. There was an energy, a health, and a movement about her. She was incomprehensibly normal and well adjusted about her body, and that enthralled me."

Linda turned out to be a Cordon Bleu–trained chef who had supported herself through high school by cooking. For her, food was not evil but an art. "She thought my whole attitude toward food and weight was stupid. I hadn't eaten vegetables in four years. I had such a restrictive diet, I was proud of myself for eating a tomato. " Rob quickly realized that he wanted Linda more than he wanted to go on denying himself—and that she would not want him if he continued to deny himself. So he asked her to help him. "She taught me to eat." She also taught him to reorganize the way he viewed the world. "I had a very hierarchical, right-wrong framework. She pushed against that in me in a strong feminist, very political way." And she taught him to fight. "We always had an incredible ability to get angry at each other and recover. I'd never had that with anyone before."

Linda and Rob married as he was beginning his medical residency. The next year Linda nearly died. An acute infection kept her in the hospital for months. The scare so shook both of them that when she recovered they decided to take the following year off to travel. "I realized the restrictive, highly structured way I'd lived my whole life made no sense. And Linda had never thought that way. So we set out to find people who were free of all that." The year was 1979. "The height of the anti-nuclear period. We joined the Clamshell Alliance fighting the Seabrook Nuclear plant in New Hampshire. We spent about six months there and met a lot of ex-hippie people who were doing fascinating service things with their lives. Then we moved to a commune on Cape Cod, a collective trying to design ways to re-verse environmental damage. We planned to stay only a month, but there was something about these people that was very attractive to us. We ended up staying two years."

Linda worked with algae and agriculture. Rob worked at a local women's clinic. They grew their own fruit and vegetables, raised chickens. Their whole household, consisting of three couples, lived on about three hundred dollars a month. "These people weren't trying to get into grad school or make a lot of money. They were growing food; they weren't rejecting it. There was a sense of personal growth here that was beyond what I'd understood was possible for me." Rob clarified: "As a rigidly obedient Jewish boy growing up in Cincinnati I'd had a very limited view of what my life could be."

I remembered the way I'd felt in college learning to dance and laugh with the graduate art students. The way I'd basked in their sense of ease—and in their openness to me. But Rob's commune experience went significantly farther. "We'd all sit around the house on a Sunday morning," he remembered, "and give each other massages. There was a lot of dancing, because it was what there was to do. A lot of touch involved in all of that, and being naked was part and parcel. Five people would say let's go skinny-dipping, three of them women—very, very, very uncomfortable for me but absolutely necessary, so I would just do it."

I know few other men who could deliver that last remark without smirking, but Rob was absolutely serious. This had nothing to do with being male or female, nothing to do with sexual opportunism. It had to do with being anorexic. When I was a child I was so ashamed of my body that I refused to use the school lavatory for fear someone would hear me from the next stall. So I knew just what Rob meant when he said, "Can I make myself do this? Do I have to put on my clothes to go from the bedroom to the bathroom? Someone else is up and out and they're not clothed, what do I do?"

The portrait Rob drew of himself in those days was not flattering: scarecrow thin, neurotic about his body, afraid of touch, intensely insecure. But when I asked what the other people in his house thought of him, he said, even now with note of surprise, "They knew I was uncomfortable, but they perceived me as a nice, somewhat shy person that they could have some fun with." Rob likened the process of discovering himself to peeling the skins of an onion. First he shed fear, then shame, and finally pretense. "I thought everybody liked who I was pretending to be, but if they really knew me they'd hate me. Instead, I finally realized, wait—everyone knows me but me!"

"I see myself because somebody sees me," Sartre wrote. And sometimes the only way to learn what there is *to* see is to ask. But the family of friends who gave Rob this feedback, the horses who served as Ruth Zimmerman's mirror, and the therapist who worked with Betsy Kelly all were objective observers who could be counted on to reflect an unbiased image. When people with eating disorders turn instead to their parents, the reflection is often more complicated.

7

TERMS OF ENDEARMENT

Family Dynamics

One's family is a precious thing, provided it's
kept at a little distance.
—Simone Weil

THE MOTHER OF THE TWELVE-YEAR-OLD was dressed for business
in a sea-green suit and gold button earrings. She had come to
the 1979 taping of this Chicago talk show looking for answers.
She had listened to me describe my experience with anorexia,
and now she and her daughter sat before me in a community
roundtable with a dozen other parents and therapists. Speaking
in a loud, emphatic voice, she leaned forward and asked question after question that pointed to her understandable wish for
a magic pill, word, or exercise that would "cure" her little girl.
Her daughter, wearing a shapeless white shirt and hiding her
face behind a curtain of blond hair, slumped down and hugged
her arms, just as understandably looking as though she'd rather
be anywhere but here. The adults pushed me to explain what I
meant by my assertion that anorexia nervosa was a quest for
control by girls who felt otherwise powerless to direct their
lives. Why powerless? How powerless? Finally I looked hard at

the girl, who hadn't made a sound, and asked her what she thought. I was throwing her a virtual microphone, inviting her to find her voice. Without hesitating a second, her mother answered for her.

When I cut her off, saying I wanted to hear directly from her daughter, the woman looked as if I'd struck her. Defensive, hurt, and enraged, that look chilled me. The girl muttered, "I don't know," and refused to say anything more.

My assumption back then, based on my readings in the late 1970s of Hilde Bruch and family systems theorist Salvador Minuchin, was that narcissistic parents—people with an inflated sense of self-importance and a driving need to be the center of attention—played a causal role in anorexia. Given the opportunity, I would have taken this girl away for a long walk, or handed her a journal or drawing pad and begged her to design a project that her mother would never see, that might just displease her mother—could the girl even imagine that? I wanted to introduce her to people who would listen and hear what she had to say without criticizing or interrupting her, to give her tools and encouragement to explore her own independent identity. Instead, I told her I wished I had written a better book for her, but maybe some of what I had put down on paper would let her know she was not alone. It was the best I could do at the time.

I realize now that my take on this girl and her mother was dangerously simplistic. Not that it was wrong. According to Walter Vandereycken, a Belgian psychiatrist who has been studying the families of eating disorder patients since the 1980s, struggles over separation and control are critical pieces of the eating disorders puzzle. Every person I interviewed pointed to family as one source of their illness and separation as one critical aspect of the cure. But researchers are only beginning to understand the various ways that families shape anorexia and bulimia. Vandereycken has found, for example, that parents of restricting anorexics tend to place a premium on appearance. They discourage frank discussion and argument and take pride in their children's "perfection." In this system kids study hard, clean their room, go to bed on time, never talk back—and if asked to describe their families, most obediently give them high marks. Restrictors usually claim to feel well loved and nurtured; everybody gets along just fine. When researchers observe these families, however, they often find things to be less than ideal. The peace, as in Gina Reed's "horror show" family, may be more of a cold silence, the love more of a demand. Other parents, Vandereycken found, send a double message by outwardly doting on their children while at the same time denying them a voice at the family table. Families of bingers and purgers, by contrast, tend to be disorganized, indifferent, or volatile. They may send mixed messages, say, by shaming a child about her weight but tempting her with Hostess cupcakes and Kool-Aid. The typical bulimic grows up not knowing what will happen next. Perhaps divorce is in the air. Or the parents are never home. Or whatever she does just never seems good enough. "I was afraid I would not be lovable if I were angry or needy," one woman remembered, "so I stuffed those feelings." Unlike restrictors, Vandereycken says, bulimics usually find a multitude of secret ways to rebel, from stealing food to sneaking drugs, in addition to bingeing and purging.

These family patterns are hardly new. According to historian Rudolph Bell, Catherine of Siena was a favorite daughter who in her teens became repulsed by the prospect of marriage. Her beloved older sister had died in childbirth, leaving Catherine with a terror of pregnancy, but no matter how Catherine expressed her fear, her mother refused to hear her. Instead, she became so intent on costuming her daughter, dyeing her hair blond, and making up her face to entice prospective suitors that Catherine felt her only way to reclaim control of her life was to pledge herself to God. To seal this pledge she undertook a series of austerities that made her unappealing to mortal men: a vow of silence; self-flagellation; self-induced vomiting and a progressively restrictive diet that soon cut her weight by half, annulled her sexuality, and inadvertently set her on the path to canonization. "Build a cell in your mind, from which you can never escape," Catherine wrote—a medieval version of the modern anorexic's golden cage.

The question is, Why do families in which anorexia and bulimia occur follow such consistent patterns? Are poor parenting skills to blame? Societal pressures? Alcohol? Drugs? Mental illness? Or does each family's dynamic inevitably reflect its own cluster of genetic traits—tilting toward chaos, rigidity, or calm, depending on its hereditary mix? Once, researchers thought that birth order might be important because it seemed that people with eating disorders were often the youngest in the family. This has proven not to be true. Nor does the size of family matter; only children are just as likely to develop eating disorders as kids raised in large clans. What has been proven true, alas, is that parents who've had eating disorders themselves often have children who are also at risk. Genetics bear some of the blame for that. So, doubtless, do family traditions of discipline and child rearing; attitudes toward status, power, beauty, and wealth. But if my interviews are any indication, another important factor is summed up in the adage: history denied is destined to repeat itself.

Betsy Kelly, the documentary film producer who followed her sister into anorexia, remembers her mother "long before Jane Fonda" exercising for hours in front of the mirror. "She would cook our meals and then not eat with us, saying, 'I was eating the whole time.' But I'd watch her cook, and she wasn't." While in treatment Betsy figured out that her mother had begun struggling with her weight around age nine, after the death of her father. "I remember my grandmother saying, 'Rose had to go to Fresh Air Fund camp because she was so skinny.' She still weighed under 90 pounds in high school." Rose recovered enough, after marrying, to become pregnant, but then her obstetrician told her she shouldn't gain more than ten pounds with each child. This prohibition had such power over her that after each of her four children was born her weight plunged back to anorexic lows. Today in her seventies Rose Kelly has severe osteoporosis and adheres to a strict low-fat "health regimen," yet she denies she ever had an eating disorder or that her attitude toward her body, food, or weight played any role in her two daughters' anorexia.

Sometimes the maternal bequest of an eating disorder is more intentional. A member of Yale's class of 2000 told me of a classmate who wore size 4 and ate little besides lettuce—and received monthly "care packages" of diet pills from her mother. Before this young woman ever left home her mother had panicked her about the danger of gaining weight from dining hall cooking. When I related this story to Kelly Brownell, he told me students who come to him for treatment at Yale's Center for Eating and Weight Disorders often feel pressure to reduce from their parents. "We had a patient once whose mother would wake her in the middle of the night to tell her she was too fat. You can't believe somebody would do that. But we do see mothers and fathers who are hard-driving, perfectionistic, and some have eating disorders themselves."

"A mother who is tormented by diet and weight," Caroline Knapp wrote, "cannot easily teach her daughter to take delight in food, to feel carefree about weight or joyful about the female form . . . And a mother whose experience of desire is based on taboo and self-denial, on feeding others and concealing her own pangs of unsatisfied hunger, can't easily steer her daughter toward a wider landscape." This can be the case, unfortunately, even when the mother understands that taboo and self-denial are singularly unsatisfying, even if she actively wants her children to *devour* that wider landscape. Joel Yager told me about a family he'd been working with at the University of New Mexico that had been fighting anorexia nervosa through three generations. Yager's patient, the daughter of the family, had begun restricting her diet at eight. She also possessed certain signal personality traits. "She was neat, the best little girl, bright, charming. She had to be hospitalized for anorexia nervosa by age eleven." Both the child's mother and grandmother had been anorexic in college, and both her mother and her father were highly disciplined athletes, ambitious professionals, financially successful. "This kid was a clone of her mother," Yager said, "but she got it earlier. She had what I call 'hybrid vigor.'"

The family's two healthy older children—boys—paid little attention to their parents' exercise and dietary regimens. When their sister was born, everyone assumed she would follow her brothers' example. The mother recognized her own history, but that self-awareness did not extend to her and her husband's effect on their daughter. "The parents were talking the talk of health and moderation," Yager said, "but not walking the walk." And their daughter, because of the way she was built and the way she related to her parents, paid more attention to their actions than their words.

So, is the solution to ban all negative conversation about food and weight? To refrain from regimented workouts? To eat and exercise only with pleasure? Children predisposed to eating disorders would likely benefit from such changes. But the lesson of Joel Yager's story is that such formulaic strategies cannot be the whole answer. Families are created and shaped by *all* their members. Just as there is no one-size-fits-all lesson plan for child rearing in general, there is no single rule for preventing eating disorders. The brothers of Yager's patient didn't follow their parents' driven example, and not every little girl would have, either. But there was something different about this child in *combination* with her parents and siblings that positioned her for trouble. As D. W. Winnicott wrote in *Home Is Where We Start From*, "For the five children in a family there are five families," and those families often bear little resemblance to one another. When researchers ask women with a history of bulimia, for example, to describe their childhood, they tend to recall more strain and coldness than their healthy sisters do, and their mothers as more overprotective, jealous, and controlling. The bulimics also, however, tend to be more anxious by nature and have lower self-esteem than their sisters. So did their families make them anxious, or did their anxieties shape their experience and, later, their memories? If my own memories are any indication, the answer is both.

For my first thirteen years my sense of family was leavened by my brother—my only sibling. Eight years older than I, he was as funny as I was serious, as resistant to rules as I was obsessed by them. Once he shot his BB gun at the windshield of the family car. As a teenager, he filled the living room with the music of Johnny Mathis and Chubby Checker. He drank Ripple and skip-and-go-nakeds with his friends and rode a rebuilt Triumph motorcycle, which he painted a color called candied tangerine. He excelled in algebra and economics, which he liked, and flunked French and English, which he didn't. I adored my brother. I realize now he balanced my world. With him in the mix I felt sanguine about my family. But when I was in seventh grade he got married and started a family of his own. I felt his departure as a jagged loss that left me, the "good" child, the "perfect student," the daughter who felt she must do no wrong. Minus my brother, my family seemed to me alien and demanding—a reflection of my own unleavened temperament. By the end of that year I was anorexic.

The genetically determined traits that each of us is born with will, to varying degrees, either resemble or clash with the traits of the other members of our family. When our temperaments match or complement one another, everyone feels comfortable. A baby whose calm disposition mirrors her parents' will have an easier time getting them to cuddle and play with her than will, say, a nervous, excitable infant. As she grows up, the calm child will "get" her parents in other ways, intuitively understanding why they have the expectations they do. She'll naturally feel close to them. When innate temperaments collide, however, the child may try to change herself in order to seem more similar, and acceptable, to her mother or father. The resulting temperamental match can become too close for comfort, just as it is too good to be true. Psychologists call this emotional act an "as if" personality. It often is very convincing until adolescence, when the child senses she must strike out on her own and take on a wider landscape. Then she becomes terrified, feeling as if she doesn't know who she is.

Age does not necessarily resolve this confusion, as I realized at a recent dinner party while listening to a fifty-year-old novelist named Gloria regale us with stories about her movie star mother. It seemed her mother had bedded and/or wedded the most decadent men of her era, from mobsters and studio heads to European princes. While Gloria talked, the rest of us devoured multiple helpings of our hostess's excellent pasta. But even as she described her eighty-year-old mother's latest caviar diet, Gloria merely picked at the single bud of cauliflower, tablespoon of salad, and quarter-slice of bread with which she'd dressed her own plate. She had strong features—a pronounced nose and square jaw—kohl-rimmed eyes, and thick, hennaed hair that fanned out past her shoulders. She wore skintight jeans and a pink T-shirt to show off her unnaturally lean body. Her mother had given her so much material, she quipped, she'd be writing about her for the rest of her life.

Toward the end of the evening, the men struck up their own conversation and our hostess, Renee, asked how my research for this book was coming. Renee was a retired psychoanalyst who had for many years treated eating disorders. After describing some of my interviews, I remarked, "One sign of recovery seems to be that you no longer delude yourself that a single Dorito will make you fat."

Gloria shot me a look. "But I think that. Doesn't everybody?"

Renee, a solidly built woman in her sixties who also happens to be an enthusiastic gourmand, said emphatically, "I don't." Before I had time to agree, the fourth woman at the party, a petite, understated poet in her early forties, chimed in, "I don't."

Surrounded, Gloria withdrew to her husband's lap, curling into a kittenish pose as Renee reminisced about her experience working in hospitals with anorexic patients. She'd become a kind of surrogate mother, she said, but the way these girls related to their mothers was to imitate them. So they did with Renee. "I remember coming to the ward, and the nurse would say, 'Your clones are waiting for you,' because every one of my patients had taken to dressing like me—and in those days I dressed in an unorthodox fashion, with sashes and scarves, Gypsy earth mother chic."

Gloria reared back in her husband's arms so her little-girl T-shirt lifted, showing off the hollow of her belly. She had badly misgauged her audience, however. The setting was suitably glamorous—a flagstone terrace bordering a lapis-blue pool overlooking the Pacific Ocean—but this was no Hollywood see-and-be-seen set. Everyone but Gloria was dressed in loose, comfortable clothes that allowed for the curves of age, and no one but Gloria pretended to be "stuffed" after eating a teaspoonful of salad.

"How are you getting along with your mother these days?" Renee asked.

"I'm all she has," Gloria answered.

It seems obvious: an eating disorder is a distress signal. When a person pretends to feel sated with three green beans, or devours an entire gallon of ice cream in order to throw it up, something is amiss in her body, her mind—and often in the emotional balance of her family. Carolyn Costin calls this the "white flag" effect.

Costin, now fifty-two, directs the California eating disorders treatment center Monte Nido. She is feisty, fit, and no-nonsense, with a lusty laugh and a zealot's determination to stop her clients from wasting their lives. As is true of many professionals in this field, her commitment springs from personal experience. From adolescence into her early twenties Carolyn saw her weight range from 120 down to 79 pounds.

She recovered without treatment, but shortly thereafter began clinical training as a therapist, which required her to re-examine the critical passages in her life. As she scanned back over her childhood, she recalled two episodes that had never made sense to her but which she suspected were central to her eating disorder.

The first mystery began with her dread of going to school in first grade. Every morning, as soon as it was time to leave the house, she would panic and cry. If left at school, she would run home. Sometimes she would even vomit. After a few months her anxiety diminished enough for her to attend school, but it resurfaced full force in third grade. Finally the school insisted that she and her mother seek therapy. "I saw one therapist," Carolyn recalls, "and spent most of the time playing with toys. My mother saw another therapist." After a few weeks Carolyn's separation anxiety mysteriously vanished, but she never understood why. So in her early twenties Carolyn contacted the therapist who had treated her all those years before. He told her that she'd suffered from separation anxiety, but it was her mother's therapy that had really helped Carolyn.

Turning now to her mother, Carolyn learned that those long-ago sessions had uncovered her mother's repressed memory of hearing a gunshot when she was very young and finding her father dead of a bullet wound. (The family story was that he had died in a hunting accident.) This traumatic event had occurred when her mother was just the age Carolyn was when she began first grade. It seemed that Carolyn's mother *subconsciously* had been terrified something similarly traumatic would happen to her daughter if she let her out of her sight, even into the supervised context of school. Only her child's immediate presence could quell her own anxiety. She'd let go enough for Carolyn to start school, but because they were so close, Carolyn continued physically to carry her mother's anxiety within herself. The mother needed to work through her history in therapy and become less frightened before the child could feel free in leaving her for school. Carolyn and her mother remained, however, extremely close.

The second episode, then, began when Carolyn hit puberty—and her father divorced her mother to marry a Chinese fashion model. Carolyn was blond, sharp featured, and big boned, as much her new stepmother's opposite as her mother was. "One day at their house, they were gone and I tried on a dress of my stepmother's, and I was too big to fit into it. I remember saying to myself, one day I'm going to fit into these clothes." Her loyalty, though, was to her mother. "My mom is a very kind, gentle soul. She never said a bad word or even raised her voice about my father's remarriage." So even though her glamorous stepmother tempted her with gifts and invitations to spend time together, Carolyn stayed home, focused on her schoolwork, and kept her mother company. Having skipped a grade in elementary school, she began looking at colleges at fifteen. At the same time, she began to diet. Within a year her weight had dropped to 80 pounds. "I wouldn't lick a postage stamp for fear it had calories!"

It wasn't really the calories that frightened her, of course. Her fear of fat was as much a symptom as her fear of first grade had been. A much larger anxiety was at play here, and the real crisis was that "I wanted to grow up and move on, but I felt I needed to stay connected to my mom." Losing weight allowed Carolyn to symbolically satisfy everyone. She remained physically her mother's little girl, while imitating her father's new wife, yet also, by paying the price in pounds, gained her independence. Eventually, when her anxiety over separating began to subside and she became more confident away from her mother, her weight climbed back to normal.

Today, Carolyn uses this story in her work with clients at Monte Nido. "The person suffering from anorexia or bulimia is the messenger," she tells them. "She's signaling something is wrong." And usually what's wrong looms as large as a tyrannosaurus in the living room. Its name is Loyalty.

"It is disloyal to everything that is not oneself if one is to be oneself," Winnicott wrote. "The most aggressive and therefore the most dangerous words in the languages of the world are to be found in the assertion I AM. It has to be admitted, however, that only those who have reached a stage at which they can make this assertion are really qualified as adult members of society." Learning to be disloyal to our parents is the normal business of adolescence. As Joel Yager said to me, "Every kid is supposed to rebel—that's your job description." But those who develop eating disorders, for a broad variety of reasons, feel they are not allowed. "I didn't want to hurt . . ." "I didn't dare disappoint . . ." "I couldn't risk angering . . ." "I was afraid to be different." I heard these phrases over and over in my interviews. Instead of becoming disloyal to everything that is *not* themselves, people with anorexia and bulimia turn their instinctive need for disloyalty against themselves—through their bodies.

An eating disorder may be only the first course—or as Karen Armstrong put it, "phase"—of this inversion. I know men as well as women who are decades past being clinically diagnosable yet still are terrified to stand up to their parents; still prefer to punish themselves through masochistic work schedules, incessant self-deprecation, even marriages that they enter into out of a sense of obligation rather than desire. In every case, there is an unspoken assumption that the truth is treacherous and better avoided. This assumption must be overturned for recovery to occur. But such a central reorientation takes both time and real courage. As Armstrong recalled the challenge of shifting away from her anorexic mind-set, "I had deliberately told myself lies and stamped hard on my mind whenever it had reached out toward the truth. As a result, I had warped and incapacitated my mental powers. From now on I must be scrupulous about telling the truth, especially to myself. I realized this would not be a popular stratagem."

Self-effacement is a badge of honor and loyalty. Somehow, somewhere, far too many of us swallowed this idea and made it part of our being. But it isn't true. There's nothing disloyal about recognizing one's own individuality or about challenging history. As Winnicott said, it's what we're supposed to do as fully functioning adults. When, instead, we maintain our loyalty to others at the expense of ourselves, we risk remaining perpetual children.

Sartre described the central principle of self-perception as the Look. We learn to see ourselves first, he wrote, through others' eyes. For most of us, at least as children, the most important set of eyes belongs to our mother. For women like Carolyn Costin and Gloria, whose mothers had trouble distinguishing their daughters from themselves, being seen meant becoming extensions of their mothers. Here, then, was the trap of perception: *I can see myself only as somebody wants to see me.* And if the inconvenient truth began to surface that the face in the mirror belonged to someone noticeably different from Mom? Well, the logical solution would be: *I cannot see myself because somebody does not—or will not—see me.*

Linda Chung was just five years old when she realized she was not the person her mother wanted to see. Linda, her mother told friends within her daughter's earshot, was "a disappointment." Linda's mother was an accountant, born in Taiwan, who prided herself on wearing the same size 6 she'd worn on her wedding day. She also prided herself on her first three children, who did their homework without being told, chewed with their mouths closed, never took seconds, and never talked out of turn. They were trim and athletic like her. Linda took after her father. She snuck ice cream from the carton. She got excited and talked too loud. Most distressing of all, she weighed too much—100 pounds at age seven! Linda's father kept himself under control by joining Weight Watchers and spending hours each day at the gym, but what was the family to do about Linda? "I was everybody's problem," Linda told me. "There was just too much of me."

Linda's mother sent her to a diet center at age seven. She sent her to fat camp every summer until she was thirteen. At the family table, Linda's "special" plate was half the size of everyone else's. "No one will want to marry you," her mother warned when Linda's weight hit 190 pounds. Finally, after her sixth humiliating tour of fat camp, Linda demanded to go away to boarding school, where she promptly dropped thirty pounds and, by college, thirty more. Five years after that, however, when she no longer even needed to lose, she began to binge and purge.

Now thirty-one, Linda sat in my living room and assured me that therapy and Prozac had helped her, that she had learned to forgive her parents, and that she finally felt attractive. Linda *was* attractive, with large dark eyes and a pert Jennifer Aniston haircut, tank top, and size 9 jeans. Yet the expression of hurt never left her face. She confided that she would like to marry but still felt self-conscious around men, that she'd like to find a job she loves but had settled for now on being a secretary. Much as she wanted to put bulimia behind her, she said, "I still feel as if I'm holding back."

I had a hunch why. "That plate," I said. "That plate they used to make you eat from. Have they ever apologized?"

Linda's eyes filled with tears. "They still think they were helping."

Linda's mother has told her she doesn't understand what she did wrong, that she was only acting out of love, to protect her daughter from a world that she believes is cruel to people who are overweight. But the message to Linda was that her mother cared more about what the world saw than she cared about what her daughter felt.

Joyce Maynard knew all about the peculiarities of demanding parents, though her mother's demands were of a dramatically different nature than Linda's family's. When she was twelve her mother was still giving her baths and sharing her bed, as she had since Joyce was a baby. Worse, as Joyce recalled in her memoir, *At Home in the World,* her mother was reading her diary, where Joyce confessed not only her budding interest in boys and her envy of her older and much more independent sister but her worry about her father's dark bouts of depression and heavy drinking. The day in 1965 after she first wrote the word "drunk," Joyce found a note inserted into the entry. It read, "My Dearest Joyce, Yes, I did look at your diary this morning. . . . Actually, because we are so close in feeling and temperament, I haven't learned much I didn't already know."

Joyce's mother never apologized for invading her daughter's privacy. Instead, she wrote, "There is no use indulging in self-pity . . . And there is certainly no use complaining, attacking, berating—or even speaking about the matter." Thirty years later, her mother's presumptuousness still confounded Joyce. "It's misguided enough for a parent to tell her child she cannot speak of her most painful feelings. But my mother goes further than that. She tells me I must not even acknowledge my feelings to myself." That's because, in Joyce's mother's mind, there was no separation, nor should there be, between herself and this particular daughter (who, unlike her older defiant sister, had a temperament that yielded to Mrs. Maynard's suffocating attachment). When Joyce was eighteen and the novelist J. D. Salinger began to call, her mother made her a special dress for the occasion and delivered her to his door. When Salinger, who was nearly three times Joyce's age, asked her to move in with him, her mother was excited. For years, Joyce said, her mother had lived vicariously through her daughters, "seldom more than now." It was Salinger who taught Joyce how to purge, to "help" her stay little-girl thin, just the way he, too, liked her.

It took Joyce decades to unravel the conflicting feelings that were bound up in her love for her mother and, by extension, for Salinger. The most painful aspect of her ambivalence, however, was the way it had twisted her behavior toward her own daughter, Audrey. Once, when Audrey was twelve, Joyce found herself reading her journal, just as her own mother had read hers. She stopped, but the violation made Joyce frantic, the way she used to feel when she binged and purged. As Audrey got older, Joyce knew she had to let go, but she felt compelled to protect her child from the mistakes she'd made herself. " I found myself looking at my beautiful daughter and panicking if I saw her turning to food for escape or comfort. 'You've eaten half that container of Häagen-Dazs,' I'd say, my own stomach tightening, and reach across the counter to put the carton away. One day I started shoveling the ice cream into my own mouth so she wouldn't eat it, all the while believing I was trying to save her."

Audrey, luckily, was different from Joyce. Constitutionally strong willed and independent, she never confused herself with her mother. Audrey didn't have the temperament for an eating disorder, nor was she afraid to stand up for herself. When Joyce, worried at her daughter's lackadaisical attitude toward the college application process, wrote her entrance essay for her, Audrey would have no part of it. "These aren't my words," she told her mother. "I am not you. You're trying to take over my life. *Get out. Get out.*"

When Joyce and I discussed this confrontation five years later, Joyce spoke with gratitude about Audrey's defiance. She envied her daughter's self-confidence and had come to admire her relaxed approach to her future and her body. Unlike her own mother, Joyce had gained enough perspective finally that she could apologize and let her daughter go. But she also admitted that she and Audrey might both have been better off if she'd gained this perspective years earlier. For Joyce, the confusion about where her mother ended and where she began had endured. To the very end, Joyce took her mother's most outrageous criticisms to heart. During one of their final visits Joyce was sunbathing and her mother critically remarked, "Did your breasts always look like that?" Joyce at the time was in her thirties, having produced three children. Her marriage was disintegrating and her mother was dying. Instead of challenging the remark, Joyce filed it away as truth, and later, after her divorce and after her mother had died, she had her breasts surgically "enhanced."

Joyce told me this story not with pride but sadness. She'd tried to imagine, she said, how her daughter would have responded. Audrey might have laughed, or she might have told her mother off. "I like to think we've broken the chain," Joyce said. "But my daughter deserves the credit."

Many of us, at least in retrospect, find that one or both of our parents wanted us to play a role in their lives that we were never meant to play. My mother wanted me to be her confidante. Part of the reason may have been that my father, like so many men of his generation, was absent a great deal. His real life, I always sensed, was at work, in the important, meaningful world of the United Nations. He left our life in the suburbs for the commuter train at seven-thirty each morning and rarely returned before seven-thirty at night. At home, he chain-smoked as he read every column inch of the *New York Times*. He watched the nightly news intently, chewing his fingernails. On weekends he went off alone to scour thrift shops or tag sales for bargains, which he packed away in his office, the garage, and a large storage hut in the backyard. Born and raised in wartime Shanghai with a largely absent father himself, my father just never seemed available. My sense of ease and intimacy with him developed out of two childhood rituals. Each Christmas the two of us wordlessly assembled jigsaw puzzles late into the night. And every spring we watched the Miss Universe pageant together.

My father's interest in the pageant was, in a way, professional. Dad was head of the guided tour service at the United Nations. In those days the UN guides were selected according to criteria similar to those the airlines used for stewardesses: in the 1960s, UN tour guides had to be single, female, college educated, and attractive. The Miss Universe pageant helped my father keep standards for the guides current. "He just likes to exercise his discerning eye," my mother would say in a tone that managed, confusingly, to pair pride and contempt. I don't remember her or my brother watching the pageant with us. I, on the other hand, curled at my father's side, devouring the show. "She mispronounced *Pyongyang!*" Dad would scoff, eyes riveted to the screen. Or, "She looks like a giraffe." Beauties with plans to erase global poverty or social injustice automatically trumped those who wanted to pursue acting careers or save stray canaries, but too much bust, too squeaky a laugh, or too vacuous a gaze, and my father would erupt, "She's hopeless!" We tried not to be biased toward Asians, but my father's Chinese heritage made this our natural inclination. We grew silent when the judges elected Miss USA or Miss Sweden instead of Miss China or Miss Indonesia. But in 1965, Thailand's Apasra Hongsakula won the crown, and my father and I slapped palms together like New Yorkers celebrating a Yankee shutout of the World Series. I was then thirteen. The following year I set my sights on becoming a fashion model. Ten years after that I became an airline stewardess. At the time, I made no connection to those evenings watching the beauty pageant with my father. The connection seems obvious to me only now.

My father's preoccupation with work left a lot of spare room in my mother's life, and especially after my brother married, she longed for me to help her fill it. We made trips to White Plains to shop for clothes, to Manhattan to tour the Met, to Vermont to hear Pablo Casals, to Wisconsin to visit her parents. These began as exciting adventures, joint escapes from school and routine, and at first they brought us closer, but as I moved deeper into adolescence I began to feel a degree of frustration that neither of us understood. I remember, in particular, one weekend the summer I stayed in New Haven to paint, when my mother prevailed on me to come away with her, just the two of us. We drove up to Rhode Island to tour the baronial mansions of the Vanderbilts and Astors in Newport. For my mother such excursions were heaven. Beaux Arts architecture! The bustling waterfront! Outlandish history! Mother and daughter together at last. My adolescence had been brutal for her, but she had persevered. She wanted so fervently to believe it was over, she ignored the way I hugged the door and stared out the car window, dissected my lettuce leaf during our sun-splashed lunch, and wandered away from her at the Breakers, fleeing gilded, bygone opulence for the empty lawns. She pretended to accept my lie that I was preoccupied with an unfinished painting.

She was trying so hard that it hurts even now to remember that day. Finding my silence unbearable, she filled it with talk of her friends and neighbors. Whose children, whom I'd never met, had recently graduated. Who was going to work for the State Department or the Ford Foundation or Save the Children. How my brother hated his new boss. Which hemlocks our next-door neighbor was felling and how that affected the view. When I still refused to speak, she confided her real concern: my father had recently retired. He was always underfoot, but still emotionally remote. Obstinate, taciturn, and brooding, he was not an easy person to be married to. But as she recited this familiar litany, I pictured my father in his corner of the living room, behind the layered barricade of his desk, his books, his newspaper, and suddenly I realized why I felt so uncomfortable listening to my mother's complaints: I was just like him.

Looking back with the benefit of therapy and hindsight, I fantasize about the conversation my mother and I might have had that afternoon. *We can't do this by ourselves. We need professional help to figure out what's dividing us, to really know and connect and acknowledge each other, flaws and all.* That's what I wanted to hear that day, what I'd wanted and needed to hear ever since I first began to shrink away from the obvious and normal pangs of adolescent distress.

I longed for therapy. Freshman year I'd even consulted a doctor at the Department of University Health, ostensibly to find out why I wasn't menstruating but secretly to see if he might suggest what was wrong with my mind. He said nothing was wrong, I just needed to gain a little weight, which was exactly what my mother said. So on we plunged, like Joyce and her mother, Gloria and her mother, and so many other mothers and daughters, fumbling blindly for a degree of separation that would allow us to satisfy our mutual needs for intimacy and independence.

Distance is not disloyal. Maybe this is why more than half the subjects in David Herzog's study of anorexia chose to physically move away from their families while recovering. Distance is concrete, like hunger. It can't be argued with. It is also symbolic, representing the geography of emotional separation. After I moved to California in my twenties, I referred to this symbolism as the three-thousand-mile rule. As long as I lived three thousand miles from my parents I could enjoy their company. If I lived any closer I felt sure I'd be submerged. This, I've found, is a common fear, even among individuals whose eating disorders are decades behind them.

With healthy maturity comes a core need to be seen as a separate, fully functioning individual who can make her own decisions as well as her own mistakes, a person who knows the difference between disagreement and disloyalty. Distance can help to enforce this separation during the transition to maturity. It also inevitably puts one's family in a new perspective. The necessary distance, as Rachel Reiland noted when she finally gained this perspective, is mutual: "The simmering resentments, the absurd game of musical chairs, my father's outbursts, and my mother's alternating grandiosity and victim's pout had not changed. . . . The script hadn't changed. The way I dealt with it, however, did . . . for the first time that I could ever recall, when my father badgered us, I openly disagreed with him. In sum, I viewed the situation from the perspective of an adult and acted like one. . . . Afterward I noticed that nearly all of them were keeping a distance from me."

I have known people who cut off all communication with their parents—permanently. In one case this set such a vivid example that the defiant daughter's own daughter eventually cut off all relations with *her*. Fortunately, permanent estrangement is not feasible for most people with eating disorders. The need to engage with family simply runs too deep. Temporary estrangement, on the other hand, can be a vital compromise.

Ella Oldman likened it to taking a vow of silence. "I didn't talk to my parents for a year. I told them I needed psychic space." She had by that point stopped using food and hunger to punish herself. She was working as a museum curator's assistant and living on her own. Still, she felt tethered. Her identity did not seem her own, and the Freudian analyst her parents had found for her did not help. So at age twenty-seven she took a break. She changed her phone number and did not share it with her parents. She quit her job and started studying to become a veterinarian. She began working with a therapist of her own choosing. The break helped psychologically. Pragmatically, however, there were limits.

"Walking home from the library one night I was hit by a drunk driver. In the ambulance they asked for a contact number and I automatically gave my father's work number." Ella's parents came to the emergency room, the first time they'd seen her in a year. Ella is moderately tall but has the build of a nightingale. She'd been hit by two tons of Chevy. When the hospital released her two weeks later, she was in no condition to return to her apartment. "The last time I'd stayed in my parents' house, I regressed, being in my childhood room. So it was hard, but what did come through is that they care about me." It was time to call a truce.

Fear of regression around parents is often one of the most persistent shadows of an eating disorder. Not even therapists are immune. "When I visit my mother, I still am at risk of dissociating," one psychologist with a history of anorexia confided to me. "I'm no longer vulnerable to anorexic behavior, but I have to work so hard to stay present and real. I make sure I pack clothes in which I feel most myself, and I phone my husband every night to talk to someone who truly knows me. *I'm actually here and you have to deal with me as a grown adult and not take me for granted.*"

The strategies that individuals develop to assert themselves are often subtle. Candace Lunt began writing letters after she realized she could never get through to her father by phone. "The receiver just never got handed to him." There were a number of possible explanations that Candace puzzled out in her mind. Her mother might be possessive of her communication with her daughter. She might be jealous of her relationship with her husband. Or she might, as the family's self-appointed switchboard operator, want all messages to travel through her so that she could control them. Given her mother's aversion to disorder, Candace suspected the latter was the most likely explanation. Alas, over a lifetime, this small, frail woman's anxiety had conditioned the entire family to behave as if she really did have the power to unplug them. Candace found that letters afforded a means of maneuvering around her mother. "It's a way for me to take the conversation off the phone that never gets handed to my dad, and if I write letters instead of saying things over the phone, my mom can't lob criticism back, because she still will do that—she can't help herself. But when I write, she'll write back, 'I love reading your letters. The last letter you wrote was filled with so much that I keep it in the kitchen drawer and I read it over and over.' For her to say that, something has shifted. But it had to shift from a distance."

With distance, sometimes, comes compassion. "I know my mom loves me," Candace told me. "She's just not able to connect with that emotion, turning thought into action the way most people do. I know she starved herself, too, as a teenager. I know she had great ambitions. She probably wanted to be a doctor, but her parents wouldn't hear of it—and she didn't have the courage to defy them. She's looked on my career in publishing so vicariously over the years. If she's been harshly critical, I now see that it's partly because she was upset that I wasn't getting ahead the way she thought I deserved to."

My own epiphany came on a visit with my family that happened to coincide with my parents' sixty-first wedding anniversary. My brother and I had never acknowledged their anniversary before. My parents usually ignored it themselves. But old age had sweetened their marriage. The loss of too many friends as well as a number of their own health scares had made us all realize how lucky we were to have one another. While they were still spry enough to enjoy it, I wanted to throw them a surprise party—a first for our family.

The celebration, my brother and I agreed, was mostly for my mother. Over the years we'd often celebrated my father on his birthday. But my mother's, just two days after Christmas, always seemed to get swallowed up in the holidays, and besides, she hated to acknowledge her age. This, then, was an alternative that would include my father, but the guests would predominantly be her friends. And instead of gathering in one of the Chinese restaurants where my father was in his element, we would rally at a local Indian restaurant in honor of the two years my family spent in India—years that my mother considered the happiest and most exciting of her life.

We arranged for the guests to arrive at the restaurant ahead of time and remain seated as if they just happened to be dining there when my parents and I entered. My mother was sitting down when she noticed the first table of her friends and waved hello, commenting that if they were eating here, this *must* be a good restaurant. Then she noticed another familiar face. Then another. Her expression went through a spectrum of changes as she registered the happy surprise of coincidence, then doubt, a flash of *Twilight Zone* alarm, and finally a rare and radiant wonder I had never seen in her before. By the time my father turned to see what she was exclaiming about, she looked like a little girl who'd just been given a pony. "I can't believe it!" she said over and over, looking from me and my brother to the two dozen friends who spanned my parents' marriage.

That night I felt decades of resistance and rigidity dissolving. As Candace said, something shifted. We had given my parents this party not because it was expected but as a heartfelt offering. When my mother thanked my brother and me, I heard a note of respect that was utterly new and delicious. This shift allowed me the emotional distance I needed to fully comprehend that my parents do not define me. For all the qualities and traits I have inherited—my father's obsessiveness and my mother's figure, to name just two—what I do with this inheritance is up to me alone.

So much of what I for years interpreted as expectation was, I now see, *their* offering to me. My mother has shared with me her love of art and nature, her insatiable appetite for literature, her thirst for sparkling conversation and inspiring company. My father has shared his passion for politics and travel, his excitement over a juicy bargain, his intellectual fair-mindedness. All of this has enriched me and undoubtedly helped to shape my beliefs and interests, but only to the extent that I *choose* to be shaped. At last I have reached a point of self-awareness and self-acceptance that allows me to care for my parents without fear that I will lose myself in the process. I do not have to be or feel like them; I have to be myself.

Today we laugh together more easily, and I am more honest in expressing my likes and dislikes, even openly disagreeing with my parents—something I would not have dreamed of doing in my younger years. This does not mean my relationship with them is—or ever will be—without tension. My temperamental inclination to shrink from conflict will never "match" my mother's more combative extroversion. And sometimes my father's dread of error looms a little too close for comfort as I try not to panic over a late tax or MasterCard payment. We are all, like everyone else on this planet, flawed, hungry, complicated individuals, and if we are to stand up for ourselves, we must at times collide. But I understand now that perfect agreement is not necessary for us to love each other. It may have taken fifty years, but I finally feel like an adult in both my parents' presence.

8

GROWING CHILDREN
Parenthood

I'm her mother. Everything she does has to do
with me.

—Mary Gordon, *Pearl*

IN A PERFECT WORLD, we would shape the lessons of our own
youth into a recipe for exquisitely happy, healthy, well-adjusted
children. Our daughters and sons would have just enough self-
esteem to weather fear and disappointment; just enough comfort in their bodies to ignore or, better yet, change prevailing
fashions; and just enough appetite to enjoy the fullness of life.
Alas, as the novelist Vivian Gornick wrote, "How hard it is to
avoid becoming what is done to us." It's that much harder to
protect our children from repeating our fate. In the world as it
is, we try. Just as our parents did, we do what we can with what
we have to work with, including not only our own experience
but also the temperaments we were born with, the culture we
live in, the resources at hand, and the people we choose to help
us. Most of us, with the best intentions, still make mistakes.
The wonderful thing about mistakes is that we can learn from
them and change.

When I became pregnant with my son I was thirty-one and more than a decade out of anorexia. When my obstetrician learned of my past eating disorder and said, "We'll have to watch that," I felt indignant. I had perspective. I wanted this baby terribly, had gone so far as to write two books on parenting and infant development by way of preparation. I understood that gaining weight was a necessary—and temporary—part of the deal. Admittedly, I did not expect to gain the more than fifty pounds that I would put on before my ten-pound son was finally born, but as long as he was healthy I really didn't pay much attention to the scale. Later, as a nursing mother it took me more than a year to lose the last of that weight, but that, too, was natural and normal. There are trade-offs you make when you become a parent, and at this point in my life I was prepared enough, committed enough, and realistic enough to make them without misgiving. One of the reasons I understood all this, however, was that five years earlier I'd experienced the shock of pregnancy—and my own reaction—when I was completely unprepared.

Back then I was still dealing with the half life of anorexia: I was sure neither that I was physically healthy nor that I wanted to be. For seven years, while my eating disorder was active, my menstrual cycle had been on hold. After I returned to normal weight, my hormones remained out of balance. As my body strained to reclaim proportions it had last known at age twelve, one side raced ahead of the other, making my breasts temporarily lopsided. My periods resumed but were irregular. At twenty-three I consulted an endocrinologist. One blood test for FSH, LH, and the other essential hormones would come back normal, the next inexplicably off. I convinced myself that anorexia had left me infertile, which at the time suited me just fine.

At twenty-six, when I received indisputable proof in the form of a positive pregnancy test that my body at last had matured, my mind and spirit still had not. My husband was not yet my husband, had no immediate plans to change that status, and

I was only beginning to work out my role as stepmother to his then four-year-old son. Another child seemed out of the question; I refused even to imagine the inevitable weight gain. For a week or two I slid back into the kind of magical thinking that had marked my anorexic years. *If I stop eating, this will go away. If I purge myself, exercise, punish my body enough I can solve the problem.* My panic convinced me finally to end the pregnancy. There are, of course, many mature reasons to make that decision, but mine was that I was twenty-seven still going on thirteen.

In the late 1990s, Harvard researchers found that the rate of abortion among women with histories of anorexia or bulimia was more than 60 percent higher than the abortion rate in the general population. This did not surprise me. Most of the women I know with histories of eating disorders, especially restricting anorexia, are either adoptive parents, childless, or have just one child. Though in some cases the reason is infertility caused by the eating disorder, the majority choose not to bear children. Chicago housewife Lucy Romanello chose faith over family. Kim Olensky and Betsy Kelly, both married to older men, were content to be stepmothers. Linda Chung, still single in her mid-thirties, doesn't want to have a child on her own.

Sometimes this reluctance leads to regret. Maureen Rader was still anorexic when she and her first husband decided to have children, so they adopted. The adoption took the spotlight off Maureen's weight and gave her a focus of concern outside herself. She gained ten pounds and began menstruating again, but she didn't think she could handle more than one child, so she had a tubal ligation. Five years later her first marriage ended in divorce. Now fifty, she told me that as soon as she met her second husband, Sean, she knew the sterilization had been a mistake. "We looked into in vitro fertilization. The process was going to be complicated and expensive. We decided against proceeding . . . but I would have loved to have had a child with Sean."

The American College of Obstetricians and Gynecologists recommends that women gain up to thirty-five pounds during pregnancy, a little more if they start underweight. For those who pin their sense of identity to the numbers on a scale, this weight gain can pose a mighty obstacle to motherhood. Another Harvard study found that the more anorexic symptoms a new mother had, even if she ate well and maintained a healthy weight during her pregnancy, the less likely she was to have a second child. A study of twelve hundred Danish women conducted in 2003 found that pregnant women with long-term eating disorders, even those who had been recovered for eight or more years, had double the normal risk of delivering a low-birth-weight baby and a 70 percent higher risk of delivering before term. A history of eating disorders also raised the risk for postpartum depression. It was findings like these that caused my obstetrician's concern when she learned I'd once been anorexic.

Fortunately, in my case her alarm was unwarranted. I, like the majority of recovered women in these studies and in my experience, had a healthy, full-term pregnancy. I agreed with Tiffany Rush-Wilson, the Cleveland psychologist who was once bulimic and now has a five-year-old daughter. Tiffany told me, "After all those years of being at war with my body, I fell in love with what my body could do." I, too, loved the mystery of pregnancy. Part of the pleasure, surprisingly, was the necessary surrender of control. Forces vastly more powerful than my will or self-discipline were in charge of this process; and for once, that was fine with me. It was even, I had to admit, a relief. As long as I knew the food and amounts I was eating were healthy for the baby, I figured the weight I was gaining also had to be healthy. And because the changes in my body were part of the pregnancy, I considered them fascinating rather than embarrassing or shameful.

"I was ready," Yvonne Anderson said of her first pregnancy when she was thirty-five. So was I. So was my friend Sally Malloy, who had been bulimic for seven years before having the first of her three children at age thirty. "When you have children," Sally said, "you have true self-transcendence. I felt very much in touch with the world beyond myself in a way I never had before, and through that I really came to love myself for the first time." Sally was not alone in this feeling. Several of the women I interviewed felt that having children finally pushed their eating disorders behind them for good. Motherhood necessarily opens up new dimensions to one's life and sense of self. When a new mother is ready for this change, it seems fitting, even satisfying, for the gain to be reflected in her changing body.

Perspective comes from knowing oneself. Knowing, for example, the difference between your automatic self—the one that reaches for the ice cream or grimaces at the mirror—and the aware self that chooses to have a baby, carry to term, and love that child with your whole being. Perspective also comes from knowing that you are strong enough to catch her the first few times she sticks an eraser up her nose or toddles toward traffic and also to step away when she is ready to catch herself. As one mother put it, "If one of my boys falls, I say, 'Get up and don't whine,' but I do hold their hands to cross the street." Knowing where you end and your child begins, a distinct individual in her or his own right, is not the sort of self-knowledge that comes easy to veterans of eating disorders, but once secured it can be a source of astonishing strength.

"Exquisite, profoundly healing, and tragic all at once." Hannah Winters was describing the stillbirth of her first child. I wondered if I'd heard right. Even a woman without Hannah's turbulent history—the years of bulimia, suicide attempts, the sordid affair with her psychiatrist that had led to her diagnosis of borderline personality disorder—even a woman with no history of turbulence at all might have been forgiven a certain hyperbole when describing a tragedy of this magnitude. This stillbirth had happened seven years earlier. Still . . . *exquisite?*

I pictured Hannah's round, soft face in the quiet at the other end of the telephone line. It was late for her in Iowa as we talked on this November night. Hannah's partner, Paula, and their two young daughters had already gone to bed. I asked her to clarify what she meant.

Hannah's voice was neither melodramatic nor stoic. After nine healthy months of a pregnancy that was the result of a carefully planned insemination, she'd arrived at the hospital seven centimeters dilated with contractions just a few minutes apart. When the nurse couldn't find a heartbeat, Hannah blamed the nurse's incompetence. When the doctor couldn't find the heartbeat, Hannah and Paula joined hands. The doctor said she was sorry, but Hannah was still going to have to birth this baby. "For eight hours I had to labor and push her out. And during those hours I had a lot of time to think and talk with the people around me. I was really clear that if Allison— that was the name we gave her—needed to leave, then there was a good reason. Maybe it was physical. Or maybe there was another mother whose baby had died and Allison's spirit had gone to that baby because the mother couldn't handle it and I could. Paula and I were so open in our grief, we just invited people to come cry with us. I probably had ninety visitors in the hospital over the next two days. We both worked for Catholic Charities, which was pretty funny, this lesbian couple working for Catholic Charities—but we had so much love and support. Two hundred people came to Allison's funeral service."

Over the weeks that followed, Hannah said, "I went through different levels of fighting for a reason to keep going. But I didn't binge or vomit or starve myself. The process catapulted me to come face-to-face with life. And when you're as connected as I was by then, the old mind games no longer worked."

Hannah's voice trailed off. The ensuing silence seemed to me deeper, stronger than where I was sitting in Los Angeles, and the difference wasn't just between Hannah's rural and my urban background noise; I felt I could hear the weight of her whole life in that pause.

When she continued she sounded serene. "This was a legitimate experience. It wasn't a drama. It wasn't self-induced. And I felt honored for the process I went through and how I was handling it, also how Paula and I handled it together. Our relationship was one of deep respect. We gave each other room to grieve in our separate ways, so I didn't need to act it out self-destructively."

I detected a note of sadness that I recognized from our prior conversations but which had not been present in Hannah's description of her baby's death just moments earlier. "For a long time I lived in other people's reflections," she said. "The slightest criticism, a raised tone of voice would tell me I wasn't okay. Then I would have to manipulate the situation, their mood, their liking, choices, preferences—I had to manipulate them to feel good about themselves in order for me to be okay."

Hannah credited a variety of therapies with teaching her the skills she needed not just to recover but to contemplate having a family of her own. Cognitive therapy had helped her retool her beliefs about what made her "good" and "okay," to question her assumption that if she wasn't perfect she must be disgusting, and to let go of her deeply held belief that the size of her body was a measure of her worth as a human being. Behavior therapy helped release her from the compulsions to binge, purge, and steal. And interpersonal therapy had helped her to identify and defuse situations, like arguments and threats, that could trigger those compulsions. But Hannah felt she'd done her most important work in Jungian psychoanalysis, a process she described as reparenting. "It was my salvation because I finally felt seen. I hungered for that. I learned that this is the most important gift a parent can give a child. But the parent herself has to feel genuinely seen before she can pass this gift on."

I wondered how Hannah had known when she was ready, as she said, to pass this gift on?

"I'd grown up thinking that to love someone you have to give up yourself, that love makes you less. Before I was pregnant, I wondered if loving a baby meant I had to make myself less—to deny myself for her the way I felt I had to deny myself for my mother, but when I talked about it in therapy, I realized I had it all backward. Loving this baby could help me gain a whole new sense of myself. I could be to my children the parent I never was able to have. Also, by that time I had more trust. I understood that the bumpy times are unavoidable. They don't mean that I'm bad or wrong. They're just life."

And life inevitably changes. Seven months after Allison's death, Hannah became pregnant again. This time she gave birth to a healthy baby girl—Sasha. Ellen, her second daughter, was born fourteen months after Sasha.

The challenge now, as Hannah grasps it, is to see each of these children as an individual in her own right, to honor their differences both from each other and from Paula and herself. Significantly, Hannah sees appetite and eating habits as mirrors of the two little girls' personalities—which are temperamental opposites. Two-year-old Ellen will eat just about anything anytime. She's gregarious, uninhibited, and full of gusto. It's conceivable she might someday develop an eating disorder but unlikely. Her four-year-old sister, however, is a born introvert. "Sasha is very sensitive," Hannah said. "She's much more cautious than Ellen and less in her body. More ethereal and much more restrictive. She will only eat pepperoni and cheese and apples, strawberries and chips at home. I don't think she gets that from me or Paula. From two months old, we were worried that she was failing to thrive. We used to howl at her: 'You have to eat or you can't go outside.' But it only made her more upset, and when she got upset she couldn't eat."

Hannah and Paula realized they had to back off and use different approaches for the two girls. Ellen they could kid and roughhouse. Sasha needed to feel calm and safe. She liked certain kinds of food in a certain order, eaten a certain way. Hannah at times would grow impatient, but she understood Sasha wasn't making these demands to be difficult; eating this way made her feel less anxious. And when she was less anxious she would eat more. "I think not needing her to be someone different than she is—that's helped."

Hannah is well aware that Sasha's personality profile makes her a prime candidate for anorexia. She also knows what she and Paula can and can't do to protect the girls. "Paula is naturally thin but recently she quit smoking and gained some weight, which is uncomfortable for her. She'll talk about how disgusted she is with herself, and I try to make her aware how the kids hear that. I'm very conscious of not making those sorts of comments about my body. Instead I'll say positive things to my children like 'Isn't my tummy nice and soft?' Or if they're a little jealous over me, I'll say, 'The reason I'm nice and rolly is so there's enough of me for both of you.'" Hannah agrees with D. W. Winnicott's description of a "good enough" family as one that recognizes and nurtures each member's individual tendencies as sources of strength. "I'm sure there are things I do that in fifteen years will turn out to be ruining our children, but if I can help them to have a strong sense of self and be able to enjoy it, including their bodies, then hopefully that will help them have the skills to cope with everything else."

There's one more important piece, however, of which Hannah is both proud and protective. "They have a mother who's done good work in therapy. And I still go once a month. It helps to have someone to just check in." This reminded me of Yvonne Anderson, who used the same term when telling me how she "checked in" through prayer or with her minister because she didn't always "trust the signals" she was sending to herself. What Yvonne and Hannah both had realized, critically, *before* they had children was that we all need advisers. Hillary Clinton may have turned the phrase "It takes a village" into a cliché, but she was right. Raising children is not a one-woman job, and the mothers who realize that and get support— whether from friends, mates, ministers, therapists, or the other mothers in their children's playgroups—are the ones least likely to backslide during times of stress into old coping habits such as eating disorders. In turn, they are the mothers least likely to model these disorders to their children.

Sadly, women with histories of eating disorders often view the need for support as a sign of weakness. Control and perfection loom so large in these women's minds that they may resist help in raising their children, preferring to micromanage their way to an illusion of power. But mothers who fear being judged by others, as well as by their own harsh internal critic, are all the more likely to confuse their children's dress, grades, soccer medals, and scholarships (or lack of them) with their own worth. Even if they hated being treated as an extension of their parents' identity, they may treat their own families much the same way.

Control is not the answer. Therapy may be. Divorce may be. But even in the healthiest families love is disorderly. Curious, growing children are often loud and unpredictable. Tired children are loud and cranky. Sibling rivalry is never neat. Being a parent means coping with the stress not only of cooking and eating and laundry but of all the complicated feelings that ignite whenever people live and love together. This is extremely difficult for introverts and perfectionists to accept. Oxford University psychiatrist Alan Stein has found that mothers who have had an eating disorder tend to be exceptionally preoccupied with their children "making a mess." They are forever mopping up after them, warning them not to spill their juice, scolding them for dropping their cereal, and taking the spoon from their babies' hands rather than letting them feed themselves. The message for these children is that food is dangerous, bad, dirty, and troublesome—something preferably to be avoided.

More sinister may be the message that the mess merits more attention than the child. Candace Lunt told me about a heartbreaking exchange she remembered from her early teens, before she herself became anorexic, that seemed to crystallize her mother's emotional priorities. (Candace's mother, though never treated, had dropped to 90 pounds during high school, just as Candace would.) "I'd been baking in home ec," Candace recalled, "and I decided while my mom was at the hairdresser, I was going to make her cinnamon rolls. So I figured out the timing, and I made the dough from scratch and let it rise, then put in the cinnamon and the sugar. I cooked these things and dribbled frosting on them. Little did I know that I'd spilled flour on the floor and there were tracks of cinnamon going here and there." Candace smiled at the memory. "I put them on a plate, so proud and eager to show her what I'd done. She comes in and throws a fit." She sighed, lifting her palms. "What are you going to do except pity the poor woman? Then, still . . . she is just canceling herself out of any kind of camaraderie with her kids. It's the cruelty of control."

Candace fights that impulse to control when she spots it in herself. She relishes the creative messes her daughter, Ruby, makes, and tries to make space for them in their small apartment, rather than discourage them. She wants to be more like the mothers with no history of eating disorders in Alan Stein's studies, who take their children's messes in stride. Without thinking about it, they encourage their babies to touch and smell and taste and play with their food. They eat with their kids and involve them in cooking. They talk about how sweet the banana smells, how red the cherries look, how cold the milk tastes. Food, they tell and show their children, is a form of sensory pleasure that everyone can share. If there's a take-home message from Stein's research, it's that mothers with histories of eating disorders need, as Candace has learned, to stop fussing and make mealtimes as well as playtime more fun for their children—and for themselves.

This sounds simple, but when mother and child are physiological and temperamental opposites, it becomes hard work. Maureen Rader suspected even when her adopted daughter, Yolanda, was an infant that she might have a weight problem. "Her grandparents were five four and one hundred seventy-five pounds. To me at barely one hundred pounds that seemed extremely heavy." Twenty years later Maureen told me she'd tried to keep only healthy—but not diet—food in the house. She never talked about weight. She walked and swam with her daughter, encouraging her to enjoy physical activity. Yolanda maintained a healthy weight until high school. Then she began to assume her grandparents' proportions.

Maureen today keeps her own weight vigilantly at 120. Yolanda, now twenty-two, is equally vigilant about her own right to look and eat as she sees fit. As an African American, Yolanda doesn't agree with her white mother that skinny women look better, and if Maureen ever slips and makes a critical remark or questions her daughter's habits, Yolanda does not hesitate to cut her off. "She keeps me in *check*." Maureen's tongue clicked with the precision of her daughter's sense of herself. "So I try desperately to keep from saying much about her weight and just love her for who she is, but it still is very hard for me. We talk about what's healthy and what's not healthy, and that's as far as I can go."

The surprising compromise the family has arrived at is culinary school. Yolanda is going to be a chef. Maureen and her husband are fully supporting her in this venture. They talk by phone with her daily. "She loves what she's doing, and she knows how to stand up for herself." Maureen looked at me and shrugged. "I wish I could have said the same for myself at her age."

Every child must eventually gain some distance from the intense attachment that bonded her to her parents in infancy. To do this she needs to recognize that her body as well as her mind is her own. Her mother's fear of fat, her mother's fear of failure, her mother's fears *for* her—none of these need be hers. It is one of the toughest jobs in parenting to foster this distance, but it is absolutely vital for both parent and child.

I did not make this up. Far from it. Having more than a few anxieties about becoming a parent myself, two years before my son was born I signed on as a writer for book projects that required me to interview such experts in the field of child development as T. Berry Brazelton, Jerome Kagan, Daniel Stern, and Dorothy and Jerome Singer. I watched through the one-way mirrors of research labs as mothers and infants cooed to each other or played with blocks. I learned how important it is to introduce babies early to the mirror, so they can see their own reflection and begin to establish a sense of themselves as separate from their parents. I watched newborns discover their own power by "working" mobiles above their cribs by means of strings attached to their hands and feet. I saw the pained responses of infants to mothers who relentlessly were "in their face," who could not seem to recognize their babies' need, even at just a few days of age, for a degree of personal distance. This research informed my contributions to *Bringing Out the Best in Your Baby* by Drs. Art Ulene and Steve Shelov, and to the American Academy of Pediatrics's *Caring for Your Baby and Young Child*. More important to me, it informed the way I approached my young stepson and, when he was born, my son.

Early on I introduced my baby to his own reflection, not as a substitute for me but so that he could get acquainted with himself. I tried to pay less attention to the ways my kids and I were alike (that was the easy part) than to how we were different, and I nurtured that difference at least as much as I did our similarities. Among the boys' differences were their physical shapes, which grew in a natural progression throughout their childhoods, from cherubic to stocky to long and lean as they are now in their young manhood. But much more important to me were their respective passions. In my stepson's case, these included building model rockets and taking apart computers, carpeting the family room with LEGO space stations, showing his little brother how to dunk a basketball, eating Oreos from the inside out, and pursuing his dual interests of psychology and digital technology as he moved through and beyond college. In my son's case, those passions included memorizing and performing songs, beginning with "La Bamba" when he was three, racing around a soccer field for thirteen years, devouring every Harry Potter book to date, making and keeping more friends in any given year than I had in my entire childhood, and eventually writing his own music and becoming a lead singer and guitarist for an alternative rock band. Weight and food were the least of my sons' concerns, and in that I was very, very glad they were nothing like me.

You could say that the defining difference was that they were boys. Having no daughters I could not personally dispute this. Megan Rainer, however, could and does. Megan's son, Geoffrey, is the child who takes after her in erratic mood and disposition. Although physically built like a quarterback and showing no signs of inheriting her anorexia, he is the one she worries about. Megan has no such fears for her daughter, fifteen-year-old Donna, whom she describes as "just incredibly together . . . and I take no responsibility for that whatsoever."

The ways Donna differs from her mother and brother are almost too numerous to count. She makes friends easily. She loves being onstage. She's on the track team and plays team sports, is headed for varsity volleyball. She's an A student who focuses on studies that interest her instead of grinding for a grade. And she thinks ahead, anticipating the major changes in her life and doing whatever is necessary to prepare for them. For example, knowing she was going to have to attend a new high school in a new town, she asked to test herself at a summer program abroad, where she was guaranteed to know no one. Through the Internet she found an international law and drama program for teenagers—in Cambridge, England. "Fourteen years old," Megan said, still marveling a year later. "We put her on the plane by herself and she went off and had a complete blast. She could go to college tomorrow and be ready."

Donna plans, but she doesn't fret. "She'll remember—ooh—it's my birthday in a month. She'll think about what she wants to do to celebrate, then she'll go upstairs and design a card and send it to her friends." Megan exhaled, recalling her own teen birthdays. "I used to think, oh my God, what am I going to do? Nobody will want to come. I want to have a good time, but who'd come? I'd put it off to think about tomorrow and keep putting it off until there were maybe two people who were free. I'd turn my worst fears into self-fulfilling prophecies and then say, 'There, you see? Everybody hates me just like I thought.'" Donna has none of these self-doubts.

Like most parents, Megan muses about where her children's traits come from. "Geoffrey is so clearly from my genetic family. Donna's more analytical and enthusiastic and expressive like her father. But wherever her personality comes from, it is a *huge* relief to me."

The risk of having an anorexic daughter was one of Megan's greatest worries going into parenthood. "Because I don't understand it in myself, and I would not wish what I've had to go through on her. But Donna, bless her heart, has a body—I wear her outgrown bras!" Donna has no qualms about this body—but Megan has to be careful not to judge her daughter by her own skewed standards. Even with the best of intentions, unfortunately, this is not always easy. "I look at her and think, if I were her, I would try to lose weight."

Donna as we spoke was five foot five, very compact, and athletic. She weighed maybe 130 pounds—far from excessive. But Megan, even thirty years past her anorexia, carried little more than that on her own five-foot-nine-inch frame, and she could not help comparing her daughter's figure to her own. Try as she might to relax her judgment, she could meet her daughter only halfway. "Donna recently said to me, 'I want to lose weight, I feel a little fat.' So I asked her, 'Do you want me to say anything? How can I support you?' She said, 'I'd really like you to remind me to eat better, because I forget.' Well, I tried to remind her, and she just freaked. So I thought, this is not working, and dropped it."

Then Donna will turn the tables on her mother. On a recent

family trip to Mexico, Megan had difficulty finding food she would eat. "I don't like carbohydrates, rice and beans and tortillas, so I didn't eat them. Twice Donna said to me, 'Why are you dieting?'" Megan sighed. "She keeps me honest."

Donna's ability to stand up to her mother likely has as much to do with her father's participation in her life as his heredity. Carl Rainer was always an active parent to both his children, but he stepped up that involvement as Donna neared puberty. One day when she was nine, Donna came to him after a track meet when the other girls were comparing their bodies, and she asked, "Dad, do you think I'm fat?" Carl emphatically told her no, he didn't think so. But the question prompted him to ask other fathers how they handled these kinds of questions. He and Donna talked about the pressure she was feeling from her friends and boys at school. They watched television together and discussed the way women are portrayed in the media. Carl wanted to teach his daughter that if the culture was sending a message that made her and her friends unhappy or sick, they should not just sit and take it but take action to stop it. So they participated in a letter-writing campaign to pressure ASKO, the appliance manufacturer, to retract an advertisement that read, "Our refrigerator is like a Swedish supermodel: it doesn't have an ounce of fat and consumes next to nothing." They won: ASKO pulled the ad. Her father's example gave Donna tangible proof that the best way to free herself from unrealistic expectations—including her mother's—is to confront them head-on.

Kyle Pruitt, who studies the families of stay-at-home dads through the Yale Child Study Center, calls fathers "the single greatest untapped resource in the lives of American children. When you look at the father style, the mother style, it's not that one's right and one's wrong. The child figures out a way to weave a stronger cloth fabric together from these two lessons they are learning." Two of the key lessons an involved father can teach his children are that distance is not disloyal and that it is safe for the child to feel and act differently from her mother.

"In normal development," Sheila Reindl writes, "a child comes to realize that if she destroys the mother she hates she will also lose the mother she loves, the one who fulfills her needs." This realization causes her anxiety and guilt, so she "tries to make reparations to her mother in the form of hugs, kisses. . . . If her mother can accept the reparations and respond without betrayal, abandonment, smothering, or retaliation, the child is able to experience concern for her mother and to take responsibility for her own instinctual, destructive impulses." And a child who feels free to express her emotional hungers is less likely to act out those hungers covertly through an eating disorder.

In a family with two involved parents a toddler learns to travel early, losing the safety of her mother but gaining the refuge of her father, which allows her to turn and go back again. She discovers in this way that both separation and connection, what Winnicott calls "excursions and return journeys," are normal and necessary aspects of life. Perhaps most important, fathers represent a sanctuary where it is safe to have feelings that Mom might not approve of, that might even make her angry or sad. A friend of mine who has recently adopted a seven-year-old girl from Nepal wrote to me of a scene within her family that vividly illustrates the importance of this polar divide. The realities of adoption are specific to this family, but the emotional interactions are universal:

> S. was playing her morning ritual of kissing her daddy and rejecting mommy (as she looks at me from the side to make sure I am sad or crying . . .). Then, when I finally trapped her in my arms and hugged her, she rejected me once more as she told me, "I don't want you to kiss me. When I am old I will not go to your house." And then she went on, "I want to be with my old mommy, I don't want any new mommies. . . . I miss my old mommy. . . ."
>
> I felt a shell cracking. After almost a year with us, she had finally put into words what was in her heart. . . . As I

hugged her, I told her how much I understood that she yearned to be with her *ama* (Nepali for mom), as I yearned to be with my mom who is in heaven, and that I would gladly take her to her *ama* in a second if we only knew where she was. . . . I said that even if she could not love me completely now, I will be always there for her, waiting for her to come to me, loving her because I am her mom and she is my daughter. . . . Tears and hugs and more tears followed. Then I told her how thankful I am that she has opened her heart to me and told me what she had wanted to tell me all this time.

Then Daddy came back and she told him she did not want to go to school today because she did not want Mommy to stay home and cry. So I promised her I would only cry a little bit inside my heart. "Yes, Mommy, but do not cry outside, only inside. . . ."

Tonight, as I was putting S. to bed, she was quite talkative, and was counting once more the friends she is going to invite for her birthday, when, in the middle of nowhere, she said: "Mommy, I like you more now!" I immediately thought to myself that it was because of her confession regarding her *ama* but I did not say anything, I just acknowledged her comment and welcomed it.

Then, as if she was reading my mind she said: "That's because we talked about *ama*. Before I liked you only a little bit, that's why I was bad with you. And that was my secret I had here."(Pointing to her heart). Then she abruptly changed subject and went back to her guest list. . . .

I was mesmerized. . . . I think that feeling I still love her, no matter what she expressed, was a surprise for her.

For all the many obstacles she faces, S. is not being raised to suppress or distort her sense of self for fear of showing disloyalty to her parents. But without that morning ritual, which placed S. in the refuge of her daddy's arms, she might not have felt safe enough to reveal her anger and mistrust of her mother. Absent the father, most children will hesitate to show disloyalty to Mother. Absent the father—or another loving, safe-harbor adult—the child may stuff her feelings down with a whole Sara Lee chocolate cake. She may starve them with a four-day fast. Or she may purge them along with the meals she eats at the family table.

If the flag goes up in the form of an eating disorder, parents need to remember that it is a distress signal, a call for help. And the earlier and more effectively the disorder is treated, the greater the chance of complete recovery. The mistake parents make, psychiatrist Mark Warren told me, is to get sucked into the spiral of blame and shame. They feel guilty, frightened, and confused, and worry that therapy will expose *them* as the problem. "But most parents are not overcontrolling; they are simply accustomed to their kids being highly motivated, highly skilled self-starters. When the kid suddenly gets an eating disorder, they don't know what to do. That dynamic is at least as common as parents who have been overcontrolling or overprotective."

Today there are specialized treatment programs for eating disorders throughout the world. For bulimia, the available array of treatments include cognitive therapy and medication which, in combination, have success rates of 70 percent and higher. Until recently, the prognosis for early anorexia was much bleaker, but a new treatment approach out of London's Maudsley Hospital may be changing that. Studies of the Maudsley method, which was developed specifically for treatment of childhood anorexia by London researchers Christopher Dare and Ivan Eisler, have found that 70 to 90 percent of patients whose families complete the program are free of eating disorders five years later. The key here is that the whole family must participate.

The Maudsley method neither indicts the parents nor singles out the child as "the sick one." Instead of focusing on what caused the problem, this treatment concentrates on the solution, in which parents play a key role. The guiding idea is that the whole family must take responsibility for making sure every-one—including, but not only, the patient—gets the nourish-ment she needs at each meal. The dinner table serves both as a metaphor for the family's interconnectedness and as the physi-cal place where emotional and nutritional sustenance is ex-changed. The Maudsley's three phases begin with parents assuming responsibility for separating the child from her illness and, with the help of the therapist, administering food as essen-tial medicine. Parents must work together, resolving their own disagreements, in order to function as healers. The job of the child's siblings, meanwhile, is to provide solidarity and help bolster her sense of herself apart from the disease. The second phase of treatment begins once the patient is out of medical danger. The parents' job now is to teach their child to assume responsibility for her own choices and health while they gradu-ally step away. Once the patient on her own is maintaining a safe weight, she begins individual therapy to help her learn how to manage the adolescent anxieties that she had been avoiding through her eating disorder. The ultimate result of the Mauds-ley method is that the whole family learns how to come to-gether but also how to safely separate.

"It's not that you're crazy making," Joel Yager emphasized when I asked what advice he would give frustrated parents. "You didn't do this to your child. Half of what I have to do with family therapy is help the parents not to feel so guilty. Everyone just needs to gain perspective."

Sometimes the perspective that parenthood brings is surpris-ing. Sometimes it casts our own parents—and ourselves—in a whole new light. But we are not merely victims of circumstance, and it solves nothing to point fingers of blame. We are responsi-ble for our own self-awareness. And we are responsible for the at-titudes and behavior we nurture in our children. Even if our distrust of food and aversion to messes is instinctive, as parents we need to learn to put these instincts on hold when teaching our kids to delight in good food and enjoy a healthy mess. We need to recognize how tightly we grip our appetites in order to relax them around our children. We need to train ourselves to satisfy our own hungers so that we do not condition our children to go hungry. And we need to learn to take risks ourselves if we are to teach our daughters to be daring and boldly pursue their dreams.

Self-awareness is not always exhilarating. Sometimes the revelations that emerge as we closely and honestly examine our families are profoundly sad. Candace Lunt told me that in the eight years she and Ruby have lived in Manhattan, her parents have never once come to visit, though they live less than two hours away. They say they are too old to come to the city, so they've never seen their only grandchild's school, never taken her to a playground or attended her class graduations. This used to aggrieve Candace. More recently she's come to see that this refusal is just another expression of her mother's terror of losing control. That terror, which more than fifty years ago fueled her own anorexia and then surrounded Candace's eating disorder, has grown unabated with the anxiety of age, in large part because it has never been acknowledged. Instead of admitting her fear, Candace's mother clutches herself tighter and tighter, pretending always to be in charge and refusing to risk making changes that might threaten her illusion of security. But in coming to understand her mother's rigidity, Candace has gained the power to reject it.

"I try to imagine the state you'd have to be in," she mused, "not to have a spirit of adventure about climbing on the train to visit your daughter. Ruby and I joke about it all the time because she wants to move to Iceland, and I say, 'Oh boy, a place to visit!' What happened to that response with my parents? I'm at the point now where I don't let it hurt me. I figure it's their own craziness. Instead, I make a mental note that in no way, shape, or form do I ever want to get to that point myself or with Ruby. I don't have to grow up to become my parents. And neither does my daughter."

9

LOVE AND OTHER TERRORS
Honor and Intimacy

> "You become. It takes a long time. That's why
> it doesn't often happen to people who break eas-
> ily, or have sharp edges, or who have to be care-
> fully kept. Generally, by the time you are Real,
> most of your hair has been loved off, and your
> eyes drop out and you get loose in the joints and
> very shabby. But these things don't matter at all,
> because once you are Real you can't be ugly, ex-
> cept to people who don't understand."
> —Margery Williams, *The Velveteen Rabbit*

HALLOWEEN OF MY JUNIOR YEAR in college brought Richard
Nixon, Eldridge Cleaver, Wolfman Jack, and Mother Teresa to
haunt New Haven. By midnight they were dancing directly in
front of me, along with a six-foot-three linebacker in a tutu and
a wizard in Prussian-blue satin. Aretha was pounding the floor-
boards of the off-campus studio where Yale's art and architecture students were partying, and the bitter air pouring through
the open windows seemed only to heighten the heat of the
crowd. I was standing on the fringes, working up my nerve to

join a conga line, when the wizard grabbed my hand and twirled me like a ballerina. Tall and long faced, with a corona of brown curls, he leaned close and called into my ear, "Your coat looks like my sculpture!" I glanced down, having completely forgotten what I was wearing: an old striped Indian robe passing for Joseph's dream coat. He thumbed himself in the chest and mouthed, "David." I yelled my name, and he waltzed me over to the Cribari, poured me a cup of wine. It seemed he was a second-year graduate sculptor I'd never seen before. Color was his weakness, he said, which was odd, or maybe not, since he was color-blind. We danced, and danced again, clowning and laughing until the party began to break up and he led me outside. College Street smelled of dry leaves and early frost. We passed the Grim Reaper and Annette Funicello doing a tango across the Old Campus. I learned David came from a place called Tarzana, named for Tarzan of the Apes. He made his native California sound bizarrely cute, a land of neon pink and drive-ins shaped like hot dogs. In New Haven, David earned money as an usher at the York Street Cinema, wore a used tuxedo to work, and named *The Last Picture Show* as his favorite movie. He told me he was adopted and asked if I was, too. He sensed something about me, he said. Something different and kindred.

The surface of David's wizard gown shimmered under the streetlights. As he walked me home he took my hand, swinging it like a lit sparkler. He described driving across country with his art materials in the trunk of his Pinto, making a new collage each night in a different motel. He used mirrors and tempera paint, sequins and glitter. Often, he said, he'd work twenty hours at a stretch, losing track of time. I fell into a similar spell when we kissed in front of my dorm room. I fumbled with my key and managed to open the door, but David pulled back and touched my cheek. He refused to come in. Later he would tell me that when he left that night he ran all the way across campus and burst into his best friend's studio, yelling, "I'm going to marry that girl!"

One pale morning in early November he brought his Polaroid to bed and held it out at arm's length to take our picture together. The resulting photo showed us cheek to cheek, the flash catching in our eyes like stars. On the back in gold marker David scribbled, "It's us!"

I didn't marry David, but how could I fail to love him? He filled his rented cottage with the music of Tom Waits, Ravi Shankar, John Fahey, Bonnie Raitt, and zydeco. His favorite author was Joseph Heller, but his reading pile included Aristotle and Tillie Olsen and Superman comic books. He wore plaster-spattered jeans, worn T-shirts, and those anti-gravitational Earth shoes that looked like they were made for Soupy Sales, but his studio was a miracle of order and polish, his tools lovingly wiped spotless and arranged like a surgeon's cutlery. His sculptures were pinwheels of color, texture, and light.

During the year and a half we spent together David introduced me to sangria at Victor's Cuban Café. He taught me how to make love in the shower. He dared me to sneak him into the dining hall (as a grad student living off campus, he didn't have a meal card), then repaid me by cooking his signature bow-tie pasta with whole cloves of garlic, irresistibly fumigating his closet-sized kitchen. We took the train to Manhattan to attend openings with Ross Bleckner, Judy Pfaff, and a dozen other soon-to-be-famous artist friends of David's. Afterward, we'd wind up at a long, loud table at Arturo's on Houston Street, drinking chianti and devouring calzones and fried clams, neither of which I'd have dared to touch in the seven years before meeting David. Now life seemed to have too much to offer for me to waste it holding back.

When the school year ended I stayed with David through the summer, and when the summer ended I helped him pack up the Pinto for his return to California. Four months later we met in Spain, where David was living on a Fulbright fellowship. We celebrated Christmas on the beach at Cadaqués, leaving a tribute of wildflowers at Salvador Dali's gate, then moved south by train and ferry and bus, consuming bread and cheese and rioja, Fanta, couscous, paella, and blood oranges from Barcelona to Marrakech. My weight had risen to 105 during the months we were in love. Classmates who never used to speak to me had told me I'd come into bloom. Unfortunately, just before I returned to America I learned that David's wife, whom I considered his ex but from whom he was not altogether divorced, was en route to spend two weeks with him.

Fury ignited impulses I didn't know I possessed. I returned from Spain to the second half of my senior year and began bringing bread, cookies, and slabs of cake from the dining hall back to my studio at night when the Art & Architecture Building was empty. *For later,* I'd tell myself, pretending I meant to work. But the canvases on the wall had gone dead. The previous year, following a general nonfigurative trend among my classmates, I'd given up self-portraits, still lifes, and landscapes in favor of large patterned abstractions. I'd persuaded Yale to sanction my month abroad with David by claiming Moorish motifs as my artistic inspiration and framing the trip as research. To fulfill the project I'd taken photographs of the mosaic designs at the Alhambra, the striped arches of Córdoba, minarets in Fez and Meknes. I couldn't look at those photos now. The freedom of abstraction made me feel as if I were falling down a well. To counter the emptiness I began to eat, and when the food was gone, I threw up in the hallway utility sink, and when I'd washed the last trace of my binge down the drain I went across the street to join the graduate painters who gathered at the Chapel Street bar. I drank Tanqueray until closing time. Sometimes in the morning I would arrive in the studio so hung over I had to go back to bed. Sometimes the drinking landed me in someone else's bed. I no longer loved the men I had sex with, any more than I loved the food I ate or the alcohol I drank or the paintings I made. But starvation no longer seemed like the answer. That, I now think, was David's parting gift, and it was substantial.

"Love," Caroline Knapp wrote in *Appetites*. "If the deepest source of human hunger had a name, that would be it." Love is identity's frontier. It's where we discover and stretch our limits, heighten our senses, engage our deepest instincts and emotions, take the biggest risks, and put our capacity to trust to the ultimate test. It's the crucible of emotion where we ultimately find out, in the words of D. W. Winnicott, if we're good enough not just to be loved but to withstand the reality that "intense loving automatically produces intense hating." Small wonder, then, that for those who feel they're not good enough, true intimacy arouses at least as much terror as it does desire.

Among people with histories of eating disorders the realm of sexuality is particularly fraught. The neuroendocrine system—that combination of central nervous and hormonal systems that regulates appetite and digestion, physical growth and development, emotions, thinking, and memory—also regulates sexual function. Or, as the gastronome M. F. K. Fisher wrote, "Our three basic needs, for food and security and love, are so mixed and mingled and entwined that we cannot straightly think of one without the others." When we deny or suppress the need for food, the effects reverberate throughout the system. Researchers at Case Western Reserve in 2004 found that anorexic patients in their twenties, and, to a slightly lesser degree, bulimic patients, have lower than normal levels of sexual arousal, behavior, desire, and orgasmic functioning. And nearly half of recovered eating disorder patients in a 1995 University of Kansas study reported "sexual discord" in their relationships.

When I mentioned these studies to psychologist Margo Maine, she seconded their findings. "Some of my patients who have histories of eating disorders are so ashamed of their bodies that to think they have sex at all is amazing. I have a patient who won't even wear shorts in front of her spouse. Sex is clothed and in the dark. For a lot of my patients, because of their shame of their bodies and their inability to let go, sex is a performance thing to satisfy the man. They do it so quickly they hardly even have time to dissociate. There's none of that, 'How can we enjoy each other's bodies?' They just don't know why they can't become more emotionally intimate."

Intimacy requires self-revelation and release. It means exposing ourselves to possible ridicule, injury, and rejection. Trust, then, is essential. When we trust another person we feel safe in his company, free to admit we backed the car into the tulip bed, that we loathe liver even when it's in his mother's favorite pâté, or that we love to be kissed on the back of the neck. When we don't feel that sense of safety, we hold back. We keep secrets. We play hide-and-seek. Orgasm, that ultimate letting go, represents a particularly untenable threat. As Judith Viorst wrote in *Imperfect Control*, "Some women, accustomed to carefully presenting themselves to the world, to always looking attractive and composed, are afraid that uncontrolled passion will expose them in some cruelly unflattering light, will show what they're 'really like,' will humiliate them. Some of these women, quite capable of having thoroughly gratifying orgasms as long as they are home alone with their vibrators, cannot have orgasms with a sexual partner, even when that partner (and maybe especially when that partner) is their husband."

When I was with David I relaxed enough to experience my first orgasm. It took five years and more than a dozen lovers before I let it happen again. Los Angeles psychotherapist Mary Kay Cocharo once counseled a patient recovering from anorexia who fainted if she became sexually aroused to the point of orgasm. "This was quite disturbing for her partner," Cocharo told me drily. "Her fear of losing control was so strong, she devised all these ways to have sex that would not be so enjoyable for her. She would have intercourse but not allow him any foreplay, for example. She would safeguard her own pleasure so she wouldn't lose control."

"Nothing makes me feel as armored," Kathryn Harrison wrote of anorexia. "All it took to relapse was my heightened awareness that I couldn't influence fate, that all I loved was fragile and impermanent: every thing, every life, even love itself." Safe within the "shatterproof glass box" of her eating disorder, Harrison felt immune to threats of loss, emotion, and intimacy. The trigger for one relapse was fear for her son, who had developed serious asthma, but her compulsive exercise and calorie counting, the tightening of her own flesh also served to deflect her husband, who told her she looked older and less attractive when she got so thin. "He preferred depression to anorexia, which he found repellent and infuriating."

Our first partners in love, of course, are our parents, so when our first attempts at romantic love go wrong, it's a natural impulse to look homeward for possible explanations. As I tried to reframe my love life after leaving David, my thoughts turned to my mother. *If I'd ever asked her advice, she would have told me this would happen. If only I were more like her, my heart would not be broken.* My mother had never openly disapproved of David, but I had no doubt about her feelings. Her silence after meeting my irrepressibly unconventional boyfriend spoke volumes. For as long as I could remember she had exclaimed over men she found marvelous, brilliant, and gorgeous. One of her favorites was an overseas IBM executive who had married a young family friend. What my mother actually admired about him may have been quite different, but what I heard from her was that this man and his wife lived in a villa outside Paris and sent their children to European boarding schools, that he could charm a prince one evening and deliver a graduation speech at Swarthmore, his alma mater, the next. What I saw when I met him was that he had fine straw-colored hair, most of which he had lost early, leaving the top of his head nearly bald. This was not a common physical type among the young men I met at Yale, but at a graduate art opening two months after my return from Spain, I spotted a candidate who came close. His family owned a national chain of hardware stores. He was balding at twenty-four, and he could quote Coleridge as he drank aquavit. William seemed pleased, even gratified, when I went home with him.

After we'd been seeing each other for a couple of weeks he drove me up to Vermont to visit a pair of his friends who were teaching art at Bennington College. It was one of those glossy sun-soaked days that prompt postcard photographers to break out the tripod and people who are truly in love to tramp up the mountain for a picnic of Beaujolais and Brie and a bone-chilling dip in a freshwater lake. Unfortunately, I'd left my camera in my studio, and I was not in love; so, instead, as William and his friends sat down to talk on a freshly mown hill, I ran ahead to one of the maples just coming into leaf at the bottom of the meadow. I didn't think; I just climbed, but once I'd reached as high as I could I found it impossible to reverse course. I perched there, dreading the moment William would come after me. He never did, any more than my mother had four years earlier when I'd staged a similar disappearing act during a party at the estate of an art collector she thought I would enjoy meeting. The collector was a friend of a friend of my mother's, an elderly man who wore a bow tie, walked with a brass-handled cane, and smiled with practiced disengagement when I shook his hand. After touring the galleries of Eakinses, Averys, Ensers, and Pollocks, I retreated to a rock outcropping, alone, to stare into the sunlight reflecting off the surface of the collector's private lake. Inside, I had refused to eat from the buffet of shrimp, roast beef, and petits fours; refused to be presented as my mother's talented, promising, brilliant daughter. I stayed until I heard the laughter dwindle in the distance, then returned to find my mother livid and hurt beyond words. Now in Bennington out on my limb, I was once again rendered mute and petulant by a role that I had manufactured and yet that felt like a lie. Only when I saw William rise to leave did I come down from my self-imposed exile.

The exact degree to which my mother and William were mixed up inside my head is no more clear to me now than the words William and I must have exchanged on the ride home that day. But I know that every time I looked at him during our month together, I thought of her. I know that on some semiconscious level I was using him to break my need for attachment. Finally I got so drunk on aquavit one night that I passed out in William's kitchen. Walking away the next morning, I knew I'd never go back.

According to St. Louis University psychologist Mark Schwartz, who specializes in eating and intimacy disorders and marital and sexual dysfunction, in many families with anorexia and bulimia "there is an unspoken fear that feelings and asking probing questions are dangerous." So love becomes idealized as total agreement—or the pretense of agreement. Yet most of us, thanks in part to Cinderella, Sleeping Beauty, and Snow White, imagine romantic love as a state in which there are *no* secrets or pretenses. We anticipate that our beloved will know everything there could possibly be to know about us. Doesn't love mean being able to read each other's thoughts? If we are to reconcile the ideal of love rendered in an anorexic or bulimic childhood with the romantic ideal by Disney, then *perfect* love must be a state of total, unquestioning acceptance that is also free of conflict. The only couples I know that fit this description are couples in which one or both people are lying.

To make matters worse, our culture teaches us that perfect love means not gaining but losing oneself. "Will you be mine?" plead the Valentines we receive as early as kindergarten. "I love you" means "you belong to me," popular music tells us. The trade-off for losing ourselves, we're led to believe, is that love will relieve us of all anxiety and insecurity. Once I become His and he becomes Mine, our problems will be solved. Thus we learn to seek a savior in a spouse. People who are vulnerable to eating disorders tend to take this, as they do so many cultural ideals, to the extreme.

But this tendency is not exclusive to our culture or even to our century. In China in 1598 a play, *The Peony Pavilion*, set off a wave of anorexic deaths among so-called Lovesick Maidens, which lasted into the mid-1600s. The play told of a sixteen-year-old girl who dreams of a lover and becomes so enamored of this fantasy that she will take only pear juice as she pines away painting her portrait. After she dies, her beloved discovers and falls in love with her picture. This brings her back to life, much as a later, Western prince's kiss would revive Sleeping Beauty. The Lovesick Maidens who followed suit enjoyed no such resurrection, however, except through the paintings and notebooks they left after starving themselves to death.

My own courtship was hardly as dramatic as *The Peony Pavilion*. It did nevertheless smack of the romantic rescue genre. By twenty-five I had recovered my weight and figure and completed *Solitaire*. I also had quit working as a flight attendant and, over the prior year, had used up my entire savings while writing a second book—a novel, which my agent advised me to burn. Despite *Solitaire*'s pending publication, I felt I'd failed as a writer and as an independent woman. That summer, when my parents offered to take me to China for a month's time out, to see my father's homeland and review my future, I accepted.

The day our tour group visited the Great Wall I struck up a conversation with another visiting team of Americans. These Hollywood filmmakers, in China to scout movie locations, invited me to join them for dinner. I gravitated to the producer in the group, a calm, take-charge man in his late thirties with curly black hair, horn-rimmed glasses, and a way of rolling up his Oxford-cloth sleeves that I found inexplicably captivating. Jewish, born and raised in the Bronx by parents who had immigrated from Russia, he introduced me to words like *baleboosteh*, *chutzpah*, and *kvetch* as we strolled pitch-black alleyways and emerged onto boulevards packed with bicycles and shoppers uniformed in Mao jackets. China came and went as I listened to his stories about making films in Cambodia and Yugoslavia and living in London in the sixties. In turn, he listened to me worry over the choices I'd face when I returned to my studio apartment in Greenwich Village, with no money and no job. Occasionally our fingers would meet. I didn't pull away. When he kissed me good night he cradled my head in his hands. The third evening we never left his hotel room.

The following month he came to New York. He solved my immediate financial crisis by purchasing the film rights to *Solitaire*, which was being published that month. We met in Chicago for a weekend at the Ritz while I was there on book tour. For the next six weeks he phoned every night. Come September he was back in New York.

My suitor took me seriously, but he also nudged me to take myself *less* seriously. He would ask, smiling, "Do you need to be fed?" and I would answer, to my surprise, "Yes. Yes, I do." It seemed as if no one had ever asked me that question before, but now that he had, I was insatiable. We'd go down to Chinatown for dim sum, uptown to Zabar's for bagels, to Spring Street Natural for stir-fry. We'd stop at Ferrara's in Little Italy for espresso, and I'd find myself swooning over contraband like ricotta cheesecake or *sfogliatelle*. He indulged my vegetarian restrictions but persuaded me to share his dessert. He wanted me to move to California. He also was fourteen years older; had already been married twice; had a two-year-old son; and was asking me to leave my friends, parents, brother, and the city I loved. We'd only met in June. By November I was unpacking in Los Angeles. Four years later we were married.

Women with eating disorders often marry older men, psychologist Margo Maine told me. "There's something reassuring about someone who's farther along in his life and knows where he's going and what he's doing, but it can end up keeping you in the same childlike role that the disorder kept you in." Eating disorders, in other words, are one way to avoid growing up, and marrying an older man another. I couldn't deny it.

Neither did my husband, even at the time. "The trellis and the rose," he called it. He willingly offered me his home, his credit card, and his encouragement as I tried out careers in magazine publishing, television news, and freelance writing. He wanted me to bloom. He liked the role of rescuer. And unlike David, he had no yen for sexual freedom.

"He's perfect," I remember telling a friend at work shortly before we married.

Twice divorced, my friend knew better. "Nobody's perfect."

I misunderstood this as a warning. It took me years to realize her comment was not about my husband-to-be in particular but about everyone—and every marriage.

"You have to write about the affairs," Pat Armstrong said when I told her I was looking at the love lives of recovered anorexics. Pat had been happily married for twenty years to her second husband but was still trying to comprehend what had driven her to the affair that ended her first marriage. "It was so unlike me!"

Pat had met her first husband while still in her teens, and became anorexic shortly thereafter. They married early in her six-year battle with the eating disorder. She had the affair three years after recovering. Even at the time, she wasn't sure why she did it. She didn't have any illusions about her lover; it was purely a physical attraction. Her then husband was a good provider. He made her feel safe—and very guilty. I asked how her therapist had explained her infidelity.

"She thought I didn't dare say there was anything wrong with my husband, so I made something wrong with me. In fact, there *was* something wrong with me. I was unhappy in the marriage, but I didn't know why, and I didn't think I was entitled to have those feelings."

"Of course not. It had to be your fault." I knew the drill. She must not have kissed him deeply enough or worn enough peek-aboo lingerie. She wasn't thin enough or clever enough. She should have listened more attentively to his complaints about that deal that went south or the Giants' fumble in the last quarter. She should have known how to make him happy, and if he was happy she ought to have been happy.

"So instead of admitting I felt bad, I acted bad."

I nodded, remembering myself ten years earlier. "Me too."

The problem in my case wasn't lack of attraction but doubts about myself. Maybe with a less self-confident man, I thought, I'd feel freer to speak my mind. Maybe with a more artistic man, I'd be more creative. Maybe I'd feel more equal with a younger man, more beautiful with a man who flattered me instead of finding me so amusing. It never occurred to me to sit my husband down and talk about my doubts, my frustrations, or my desires. I dreaded conflict and was afraid he would be offended or angry if he knew what I was really feeling. Instead I kept my antennae up for men who were younger, more intellectual, more aesthetically sensitive. If the right one came along, I wouldn't rule him out. Twice I thought the right one had . . . for about forty-eight hours each time.

After the second, I tried to tell my husband that something was wrong, but I couldn't articulate what and burst into tears. By then, though he didn't yet fully know why, he was fed up. Slamming his hand on the dining room table, he gave me an ultimatum. "Just make up your mind. Are you in or are you out?"

I secretly consulted a therapist alone, still not daring to suggest marital counseling. She said, "I guess you don't have the kind of marriage that would allow you to tell him you'd been attracted to someone else."

"No!" The very idea panicked me. Instead of confessing, I made up my mind. I was obviously the problem, so I would do whatever it took to make the marriage work—with one exception: I could not tell the truth.

Five years later, under the stress of a doomed business venture that had been working him twenty hours a day for more than three years, my husband turned on me. He referred to me without irony as his "ball and chain" and, in one surreal spasm of rage, as "the hound of hell." Later, reviewing this uncharacteristic cruelty in Dr. Gold's office, he claimed that his rage was directed at me, "because you were closest."

This was doubtless true, but I was guilty of far more than that. According to the implicit system of our marriage, my crime had been my failure to rescue my husband in his time of need as he had once rescued me. He needed a personal assistant, a saleswoman, a marketing manager, a financier, and a fairy godmother, and I was only his wife. I'd learned over our years together how to write a novel, raise two boys, make a home, and be a cautious companion, but I had no idea how to be honest with him, much less how to save his business.

Unfortunately for my husband's business, no one knew how to save it. Once the company had folded, however, he began to reassess not only what he truly needed but what he'd been striving so hard to achieve. He had never been and would never be an all-powerful Prince Charming. I surely was no Sleeping Beauty. I could no longer pretend that his kiss was all it took for me to be happy, and he had long ago shed his desire for an ornamental wife.

We both needed more—more truth, more trust, more disagreement, more excitement, and more compassion. If he wanted to stay in business, he was going to have to build a company that required human rather than heroic efforts. And if he and I wanted to stay together, we were going to have to build a partnership that didn't put either of us up on a trellis—or out on a limb.

D. W. Winnicott wrote that people who feel threatened by love assume that intimacy means "living in a world which is really created by the other." This assumption gives one's partner in a relationship all the power, creativity, and freedom, whether he wants it or not. The less-powerful partner feels she must either disappear, becoming wholly selfless, passive, and subservient, or else she must deceive, concealing her true self. In either case, Winnicott writes, there is usually, "a compulsive element in it all, and this compulsive element has fear somewhere a long way at the back of it." Fear of failure. Fear of rejection or abandonment. Fear of being exposed.

To turn such fear around, Sheila Reindl told me, we have to stop acting and thinking of ourselves as passive objects of desire. "I talk to patients about what it means instead to be a *subject* of desire. Sexual desire. Desire for comfort." A participant in rather than a recipient or victim of love.

The lesson does not always come easy. Reindl said that several of her patients, after avoiding men for years, developed a compulsive need to be adored. Typically, however, the high of adoration was short-lived. "The feeling in the moment is so good," Reindl explained. "But this adoration seeking can lead to a cycle of ended relationships because neither party has a full appreciation of or investment in the other." Laugh a little too loud, show your sulky side, or turn up at dinner with your hair still wet, and it's easy to lose your footing on the pedestal. There's just not much room up there for error or honesty.

The same syndrome can work in reverse with similar results. As Ella Oldman said, "Part of the anorexia that lingered was that incredible need to be loved. And yet nothing is enough. People could move mountains for me, but if they failed one test, I couldn't really trust them anymore. Prove to me that you love me, and you have to be infallible in that test." That test, of course, becomes an insurmountable obstacle rather than an entrée to love.

Another typical solution is to accommodate emotional cynicism by selecting a mate who doesn't want to get too close. In 1995 researchers at the Flemish Institute for Health Promotion in Brussels, Belgium, videotaped sixty-three couples to see if women with eating disorders interacted differently with their husbands than did other women. Sure enough, compared to healthy couples, those with eating disorders showed less intimacy, less constructive communication, and less openness. They didn't fight, and they didn't belittle each other, and they didn't say they were unhappy. They just weren't particularly close or engaged. "I would say a lot of my patients are in that kind of relationship," Margo Maine told me. "These marriages can sometimes last forever. The guy may find intimacy other places, but a lot of them are just not capable of intimacy."

"I don't want to be intertwined with someone," one former anorexic told me. "I need a lot of space and to not have to tell him everything I'm doing. And he doesn't want to know everything I'm doing. He really is the ideal guy for me." Another put it this way: "It's there in my mind that there's a piece missing, but I think I've sewn the tapestry around that. Sexually, I never really opened up." Others, like forty-four-year-old Andrea Wiley, reserve their unqualified affection for partners they know will never challenge them. Throughout her twenty years of marriage, no children, Andrea told me, she has lived "at a slight remove from my husband to avoid ever being hurt. My love for my golden retriever, however, is so deep that I fear for myself when her time finally comes. I feel such joy because of her and I feel guilty that I know I love her more than my husband. I tell myself that it's because of her innocence, like a child. So that's why my love for her is so much more intense than my love for my husband. But I think it's really because I don't want to feel anything that intense for another human. It's too dangerous and scary."

Such arrangements preserve each partner's sense of control and reduce the risk of conflict, but, as Andrea recognized, they also reduce the possibility for deep human connection. This may help to explain how some wives can binge and purge for years without their husbands noticing, how others can suddenly drop to 100 pounds and spend four hours a day on the StairMaster without their husbands becoming concerned. "Instead of loving each other," Erich Fromm writes of partners in this kind of marriage, "they settle for owning together what they have: money, social standing, a home, children." The problem is that, sooner or later, one of the partners may sense that, for all their possessions, something vital is missing.

"I think of anorexia as her survival suit," Mary Kay Cocharo said of the woman I was about to meet. "She's been in recovery for many, many years, but she still has behaviors that keep her very tightly controlled, and that affects intimacy. The ways in which she's willing to have sex and the ways she's able to climax are very limited. Jill's husband loves her very much, but he feels he has given up a lot of passion in his life in order to be with her because she's so controlling. It goes way beyond what food she eats." Cocharo had been Jill and Ed Jameson's therapist on and off for more than twelve years. When she invited Jill to meet me, Ed encouraged his wife to be interviewed. He thought that talking about her old anorexic habits might help her understand some of his concerns about their sex life.

We met in Cocharo's office. Jill looked like a model for Ann Taylor. Her slacks were tailored, her sleeveless blouse pressed. She wore her hair frosted and expertly blunt cut and, judging from her sculpted arms, worked out daily. I guessed her age as late forties, though her figure suggested a decade younger. She gave my hand a firm shake and hurtled into her story. She'd always been self-conscious about her weight, she said, even though she was never actually overweight. "My two brothers and sister made fun of my body from the time I was about five years old. When my stepfather heard them, he said, 'No, those are the best parts.' Then he would pat me on the rear. I saw him do that to my mom but not to my sister or anyone else. And every time he kissed me he would use his tongue."

My gasp startled her. But then she seemed to feel the need to apologize. "Not that I had any sense what that was about."

This struck me as an odd disclaimer. Would it have been worse if she *had* understood what he was doing? I wondered if she feared I might think she'd asked for these kisses. "Did you tell your mother what he was doing?"

Jill shook her head. "They had their own problems and I didn't want to go there. I guess I never could figure out whether it was right or wrong. It didn't feel right, but I just didn't know."

"There's the question of, 'Why not tell Mom?'" Cocharo said. "There's also the question of, 'Why not confront him?'"

Now Jill gasped. "Oh no! I could never have done that."

Instead, when she was fifteen she escaped the problem by shrinking herself until her stepfather no longer came on to her and her siblings stopped teasing her. Five feet three inches tall, Jill dropped to 82 pounds over three years. She still weighed less than 100 when, at twenty, she married her college sweetheart. Later that year, Karen Carpenter died. Jill was a fan, had been to a Carpenters' concert just a few months earlier, and was shocked into action by the singer's death. First, she went shopping for clothes with elastic waistbands, "so I could expand and it wouldn't be so in my face." She began therapy and, though it took five years, put on ten pounds.

Jill's need for control in other aspects of her life, however, was less flexible. She might have to gain weight, she reasoned, but she didn't have to get fat. Others might have followed this reasoning to take an aerobics class once or twice a week. Jill became an aerobics instructor. After taking over the family finances she would set aside whole days to deal with bill paying, accounting, and taxes. In her free time she alphabetized her spices, reorganized her Rolodex.

Cocharo shook her head. I had to laugh. Jill looked at me.

"I used to do that," I said.

"I never did." Mary Kay Cocharo, a woman of middle age and normal weight, had never had an eating disorder. Like Jill, she was dressed in a casual top and slacks, but unlike Jill, who managed a large real estate office, she hadn't bothered to brush her hair or apply lipstick, powder, and eye shadow before our meeting. She actually looked as if she'd been hard at work on this hot summer day.

The way Cocharo put it, she was a "maximizer," someone who reacts outward, making more of herself in order to command attention, while Jill and I were "minimizers," who withdrew, backed up, or pulled inward to avoid unwanted attention. The significance of calling people with histories of anorexia minimizers was not lost on me.

Jill suspected that her tendency to shrink from attention was related to her ambivalence about sex and pleasure. "I do remember when I was in high school, before becoming anorexic, I enjoyed foreplay." But later she wouldn't allow herself that feeling. Instead, she forestalled even the possibility of sexual pleasure by marrying a man who did not arouse her. As she regained her physical health, however, her desire for sexual pleasure returned and with it a certain torment. Did she or didn't she deserve satisfaction? Was it good or bad to want it? Why did she still not feel this desire for her *husband*? "I remember thinking, What is going on here?" Jill proposed couples therapy. Her husband refused. She asked for separation. He countered with divorce.

In characteristic fashion, Jill set about her search for a second husband through the safest, most organized, and least messy method she could imagine: a dating service. "I wanted to have some research done so before I met him I could read about him." Ed's listing said he'd been married once, divorced for five years, and worked as a business consultant. Also, while at Stanford, he'd studied in a Buddhist monastery. "And the picture he chose for the album was taken at a child's birthday party. He had a clown nose on and a big hat." Fortunately, when he met her for lunch he left the clown nose home, and she discovered he had a rugged cleft in his chin, broad cheekbones, deep-set blue eyes that never seemed to leave her face—and that he excited her in a way her first husband never had.

Jill thought marrying a man she found sexy would resolve her inhibitions. But her stepfather kept showing up in bed with them. "To this day I still have to say, this is my husband approaching me, not my stepfather. I have a hard time saying, 'Don't do that, it doesn't feel good.' That's what I never could say to my stepfather."

"And what about, '*Do* do that, it does feel good'?"

"Just starting to get to that one!" She looked at her therapist and sighed. "How old am I, fifty?"

Cocharo spoke quietly. "In relationships people are kind of in a circle with a fence around them, and whenever we open an exit door we dilute the intensity and the intimacy of the relationship. We all have exit doors. They can be very benign or quite positive, like taking care of your children or having a big career. It doesn't have to be alcohol or sexual addiction or suicide or affairs. I think Ed would say that some of your old anorexic patterns have served as exits."

"Like what?" I looked first to Jill, but she waited for Cocharo to speak.

"I think one of the disappointments for him is that he's more social and he loves to have people over spontaneously and cook dinner. For Jill that creates a lot of anxiety. She wants a lot of lead time. She wants to clean the whole house. She wants everything to be—"

Jill and I finished Cocharo's sentence in unison: "Perfect!"

Jill took off her glasses and folded them in her lap. "I think when he says a part of the anorexia is still there, he's referring to our sexual life. He's very frustrated. Disappointed in what we've lost as a couple sexually, what we could have experienced. Or the pleasure that he thinks I'm not getting. He's voiced many times his disappointment that I was not interested in different positions, being more adventurous. I didn't realize that was a controlling thing, just being in one position during sex. I never put that together. Now we do talk about it. How was the last sexual experience, and what do we need to do next time?—that sort of thing. I'm a little more open to that now. He's always been open to it."

"What about other aspects of intimacy?" I asked. "In terms of being able to talk about things that bother you, fears, or if he's doing something that upsets you, can you confront him?"

"Mary Kay has helped us with that tremendously. I wouldn't hesitate to have that conversation now at all. Sometimes I actually think I'm nagging him."

"I think he's waited so long to hear from you," Cocharo said, "now you think you're being a nag and he's thinking, Yes! Tell me how you feel."

*   *   *

When my husband and I sat down for counseling, Dr. Gold wanted to know about the good times. "If you start new you have the option of picking and choosing from the past. So tell me if there's anything you'd relive if you could go back in time."

My husband responded as if to a verbal Rorschach: "Margaritas and mud pies."

I felt myself blush. We were in our final stage of separation, "dating" several times a week as we tried to decide if we'd finally had too much of each other, and here he was recalling a time when we couldn't get enough . . . of anything. We'd been entirely different people back then, but Gold's eyebrows shot up, his Groucho Marx imitation. He turned to me for elaboration.

"Our hedonistic phase," I explained. "The first couple of years after I moved to LA we were living in Westwood, walking distance from the UCLA track, the bar at Acapulco, and Häagen-Dazs. So we'd go running every morning for an hour, and every evening we'd drink margaritas until we felt silly and then bring home a mud pie."

"And fall into bed." My husband sighed. "Straight to dessert, no dinner, no rules."

"We both gained a lot of weight that year."

"Did you care?" Gold asked.

"No."

"Were you happy?"

We answered in unison, with a little coda of shock. "Yes!"

Gold folded his hands over his belly and gave us a stern look. "Mud pies and margaritas," he said. "Remember that."

M. F. K. Fisher once reminisced about her husband Dillwyn Parrish: "We celebrated with the first of ten thousand completely enjoyable drinks. Everything was all right after that, for as many more years as he was on earth, and I lived secure and blessed for those years, too, through many terrors." Gold believed in a similar standard. Some had days of wine and roses. We had years of mud pies and margaritas. He was convinced our formula meant we belonged together. It took a few more months for him to persuade us that he was right, but gradually, as our dates lengthened into weekend picnics at the beach, flights to the south of France for rosé and *pistou* in medieval hill towns, and to Dublin for bangers and ale, we began to come to our senses. We shared not only sex and Prosecco, but movies and boxes of Dots. We shared memories of the Great Wall and our long-distance courtship; of our three-year-old singing Guns n' Roses' "Take Me Down to Paradise City"; of the darkness after the Northridge earthquake when we flipped through family photo albums by candlelight to stay calm. We had mornings now when, once again, my husband and I lay in bed for hours concocting imaginary *Saturday Night Live* skits or arguing over U.S. policy in Afghanistan or exploring each other's skin. We sang "The Teddy Bears' Picnic" in the bathroom and "A Real Nice Clambake" in the kitchen. None of this was new. We'd had these songs, this play, this pleasure in each other all along. Only one critical component had been missing.

"Honor." The first time Dr. Gold introduced this word I felt as if a tidal wave had crashed inside my head. Of course I knew intellectually that to honor meant to esteem, to show respect and regard, to value, to accept and care for deeply. But somehow, many years earlier, this word had become entangled in my mind with threat. Doubtless the phrase "to honor and obey," which was stamped into the psyche of every growing American girl before the advent of *Ms.* magazine, had something to do with this. To honor and obey—a pledge typically reserved for brides, soldiers, and children—implied submission.

I went home from that session and checked our wedding vows, which I'd taken primary responsibility for scripting back in 1983. Sure enough, we had pledged our mutual love and re- spect, protection and comfort, to be "equal partners in life," but I'd banished the word *honor* from the ceremony, as well as the pernicious *obey.* I stared at the typewritten sheets now, the last of a dozen revisions over which I remembered laboring for months and considered how much more than semantics had been at stake. I hadn't just omitted a word; I'd balked at a cen- tral principle of life. Moreover, I'd done this *throughout* my life. If I honored my parents, I sensed as a child, I'd be giving in to their power over me. If I honored my body, I told myself at four- teen, I'd be surrendering my willpower to physical weakness. If I honored my age, I'd abandon my youth. And even as I raged against separating, that automatic pilot inside my head had warned that honoring my husband meant he'd win and I'd lose. The fallacy of my thinking about honor was like that of a child who fears her mother will love her less when her sister is born. As if honor were a finite commodity that must diminish in both quantity and value if given away. In fact, the opposite is true.

"There was one moment in particular," I said at our next ses- sion with Gold, "when I began to realize my mistake. I just never applied the word *honor.*" I was referring to a Chinese ban- quet my husband had thrown for me in 1994 as the publication party for my first novel. We'd rented a private room in the Em- press Pavilion in LA's Chinatown and invited all our personal friends, business acquaintances, and anyone else we knew who might have a professional interest in the book that I'd devoted five years to writing. Courses of bitter melon, glazed duck, steamed crab, and minced pork rolled out in succession as I circled the tables, working up my nerve, smiling until my face stiffened. Finally I stood up to speak. I thanked the members of my writing group, saying they really deserved the credit for any merit the book possessed. I acknowledged my editor and publisher and agent, who had refused to give up on me even when I delivered a first draft so muddled they couldn't tell whether it was a murder mystery or a historical romance. I said something nice about the restaurant, which served all the dishes I wished I'd learned how to make growing up with a Chinese father—but then, I was so hopeless in the kitchen I couldn't even boil an egg. It was one of those classic displays of self-annihilation that left me shrinking into a seat on the fringes of the party, wishing for a wand that would transform me into someone—anyone—else. A few awkward minutes passed after I stopped. Then a friend of ours stood up, a woman director from New York who had been married for many years to her Japanese business partner. "I've been around long enough," she said, casting me a disapproving glance, "to know that behind almost every great woman stands an exceptional man. And in this case, he's one of the best." She raised her glass and toasted my husband.

"She was right," I told my husband in the therapist's office. "I've never forgiven myself for not honoring you that night." My voice began to shake. "I had no idea what the word even meant."

My husband put his arms around me, and suddenly I was sobbing. He took my face in his hands. He hadn't even thought about it, he said. He kissed me on the forehead and then on the nose. Slowly, deliberately, he kissed each cheek.

Gold slipped from the room. Later he would tell us this embrace was the beginning of our second marriage.

Part Three

A WIDER WORLD

Consumer Society and Body Image

10

CONSUMING PASSIONS
Competing for Health

I saw green
for the first time in years—

it blinked from hickories,
hummed an obligato
under the wind's melody;
it smelled like horses,
new love, and opening.

It tasted like health
I was not ashamed
to stuff it in my mouth
and let it stain my words

green.
—Leslie McGrath, "Green"

EVERY EVENING AT EIGHT O'CLOCK a middle-aged woman hobbles past our house like a specter of my former self. She wears leggings and sweats, her fading hair drawn up into a ponytail that shivers as she drags her body, always alone, up the middle of our low-traffic street where the lights minimize threatening shadows and the pavement is flat. Five years ago, when I first moved here, this stranger (who for reasons unknown commutes to our neighborhood, parking down the block during her workouts) jogged upright in brisk, determined strides. Then she began favoring one ankle and racewalked, stopping often in evident pain. Now she moves in a caricature of fitness, her gait crablike, her face pinched, her pace just ahead of a crawl. Yet if one night I went out and asked why she subjects herself to this punishment, I have little doubt she would tell me she does it for her health. That was always my excuse.

"I remember you going out to run every morning," my friend Demetre told me recently, recalling the days when she lived next door to me in New York. "It was clear to me it wasn't for fun or exercise. It was compulsive." Demetre had worked on Wall Street in her twenties, surrounded by people who were compulsive—in getting ahead, moving up, proving that they were the fittest and strongest and most in control of their money, their firms, their looks, their status, all of which they, too, insisted was healthy and good. Demetre, however, quit her brokerage firm in her thirties to become a weaver. She supported herself by working at the Museum of Modern Art. Later she worked alongside her first husband in his furniture design firm. After his death, she learned the art of gardening and worked alongside her second husband, who owned a nursery. Recently she's added painting to her creative pursuits and, in her spare time, works for land conservation. "I always wondered why you were so hard on yourself," she said to me. But back when we were neighbors I made sure neither Demetre nor anyone else got close enough to ask me that question.

I began running in my twenties with one ankle already weakened from a bad sprain I'd failed to tend to properly in college. I was never fluid or easy on my feet, and, except for the endorphin high that would kick in at about mile three, I never enjoyed jogging. I did it to pay for the weight I'd gained. I did it to brake the gain. In the early years of my marriage I also ran to compete with my husband, or at least to prove that I could keep up. When I began to question our relationship I took off alone, running marathon distances, three or four hours at a stretch. But far from questioning my commitment to an activity I didn't enjoy, I prided myself on my endurance and discipline. I expected others to admire me for it, just as they had when I lost thirty pounds in junior high school. When I mentioned my new "passion" at work, however, one astute colleague at NBC instead replied, "I'm sorry." Though startled, I didn't dare stop to consider what she was trying to tell me.

I repeatedly strained both ankles and ran through the pain. In the meantime, I remained a vegetarian, as I had been since my anorexic years. No red meat, no fat, no salt, little dairy, rarely chicken or fish. (I was not then underweight; this was all supposedly for my health.) In my fifth month of pregnancy I quit running and began swimming timed laps. After giving birth I developed one sinus infection after another. I responded by adding aerobics to my swimming regimen. I began to feel light-headed, was chronically exhausted, and had trouble focusing well enough to drive. I consulted a nutritionist, who prescribed red meat. Finally I surrendered.

For years I'd been telling myself and anyone else who cared to listen that I "could not" eat meat. I claimed the enzymes in my stomach would rebel. I said all that protein would make me gag. I associated with hamburgers the same disgust I'd once leveled against my own body. If these fear tactics had the slightest truth to them I would surely remember the traumatizing or sickening or painful experience of eating my first steak in twenty-two years. But as far as I can recall there was no discomfort. In my usual zealous fashion, I had red meat three times that first week and, to my husband's amusement, enjoyed it. The sinus infections, fatigue, and dizziness were gone in a matter of days and have not returned in the seventeen years since. My return to meat had no effect on my weight, but I did find that my concentration improved and I no longer craved sweets, so my consumption of sugar plummeted.

Health was not all I regained. I rediscovered the sweetness of lamb with mint jelly, the snap of horseradish on rare roast beef, the jewellike taste of salty prosciutto wound around a fresh fig. I developed a new admiration for the writing of epicureans M. F. K. Fisher and Ruth Reichl, who once described foie gras as "little explosions on the tongue." I found myself experimenting with sections of *Joy of Cooking* that I hadn't even opened since I was twelve. And I became a vastly more appreciative— and welcome—guest at dinner parties. The damage to my right ankle, however, was less reversible.

At some point during all those years of pounding and restricting, of failing to respect my body's message of physical pain, the blood supply to my right talus, the central anklebone, had been severed. This caused the bone to die, a condition called avascular necrosis. When the damage prevented me from walking, let alone running, surgeons attempted a graft. The procedure was only partially successful, leaving me with chronic pain and a joint with limited motion. My body had finally forced the message over my stubborn will: I could walk, but I could not run.

I was forced to remember that I love to walk. I love the leisure of it, the freedom and ease of moving and looking, breathing and listening. During the long walks I used to take growing up in Connecticut I would watch the patterns sunlight made in the canopy of leaves overhead. In Manhattan I would search for the nineteenth-century busts, leering gargoyles, and Art Deco flourishes tucked under the rooflines of skyscrapers. At the beach I would notice how the surf kept time with my breathing, how the sand yielded differently beneath my feet if I curled or stretched my toes. I now realized, yet again, that my compulsion to do something that hurt me had very nearly cost me the freedom to do something I genuinely loved.

My postanorexic compulsions were typical of people with histories of eating disorders. Kathryn Harrison, for example, reflects in *The Mother Knot*: "During the years after I'd weaned my son and before I was pregnant with our second daughter I'd managed to keep my eating disorder mostly in check. Afraid of setting an injurious example for my older daughter, I'd willed it into less objectionable compulsions, with less observable effects. I'd been a vegan. I'd been a health crank. I'd fixated on carrot juice and non-genetically modified soy." In fact, people so commonly phase from eating disorders to vegetarianism that one therapist devised a test to gauge her patients' motives. She asks what animal rights group they belong to. When they can't answer, she knows "It's just another way to justify restriction." Exercise, too, is a form of restriction. Kathryn Harrison ran "ten miles a day depending on garlic supplements to protect my joints as I spent enough cartilage to purchase knee surgery." Jane Fonda created her famous Workout less than a year after she stopped bingeing and purging. It took her years more to admit that she was still "way too compulsive when it came to exercise."

The forms of exercise that replace anorexia and bulimia can look merely overzealous, or they can seem bizarre. UCLA psychiatrist Deborah Lynn told me about a rare movement disorder one of her patients developed while recovering from anorexia. With each regained pound the woman became more tense. By the time she'd reached a normal weight she was holding herself so tightly she could move only in slow motion. Lynn's story didn't seem so strange to me, however, when I remembered an incident that occurred while I was recovering from my ankle surgery. My physical therapist, a lanky woman, as I recall, with abundant untethered curls, wanted to see me walk. I stuck my hands in my pockets and started toward her.

"What are you afraid of?" she asked. "Relax. Swing your arms. Walk naturally." She thought I was being tentative because of the damage to my ankle, but I always walked with my hands in my pockets or clutching the strap of my purse or folded under my arms. This was the first time I'd ever realized how strange it felt for me to move in a way that other people considered natural—by letting go. I've been consciously "naturalizing" my walk ever since.

In some respects compulsion and passion are easy to confuse. Both consume substantial amounts of time and energy. Both command undivided attention. Both typically lead to tangible results that we believe will make us feel fitter, happier, and stronger. But as Kim Chernin observed in *The Obsession*, the compulsions that surround and succeed eating disorders *suppress* precisely "the qualities of which greatness is made: passion and vision, a wild ambition, a powerful social awareness, an overpowering thirst for learning and development, an impassioned love of life, a great gift for expression." Passion, unlike compulsion, makes us feel both good and good about ourselves. Passion makes us want more. Even its language is expansive—we speak of people who are *hugely* passionate, who have *large* dreams, *great* ambitions, *sustaining* desires. But when passion is replaced or overtaken by compulsion, it inevitably shrinks back into anxiety.

The confusion is compounded by corporate culture and the advertising industry, which seem to make ever more aggressive attempts to commodify passion into products or trends that we must compulsively own or consume in order to feel better. If depressed, we need only join Jenny Craig, purchase a Cadillac, or take a trip to Maui. Buy a new iPod or Calvin Klein jeans, and we'll forget we hate our job. Wear Prada shoes, and we'll feel like Somebody. And a new house with a swimming pool in the "right" part of town might be just the solution for a troubled marriage. "This is the seduction," Caroline Knapp wrote in *Ap-*

petites, "the velvety promise of consumer culture—*fix what ails with a product; look outside the self.*" This seduction is only a slight variation on the promise that we can fix what ails us by shaping a perfect body, and so those who fall prey to the body myth tend naturally to fall for the come-ons of commercial— and competitive—consumption. Deborah Lynn told me of one former bulimic now in her late forties, married with children and a high-powered job, who changed her fashion style, hairdo, car, fitness regimen, social set, and even spiritual practices every few months. She had stopped purging in her mid-twenties, but without treatment her other habits of consumption had become even more compulsive than her eating disorder. "Everything was on the surface," Lynn said. "That kind of hyperactivity is a form of denial. She's forever taking in and spitting out, and nothing ever gets fully digested or absorbed. But it sucks up all her attention, so she can never dig down underneath and look at the fear that's really driving her."

Kelly Brownell, whose book *Food Fight* traces the link between the food industry and America's health and weight problems, told me his research shows our consumer compulsions fuel both eating disorders and obesity. Even if 60 percent of the factors that cause eating disorders are genetic in origin, he said, that still leaves 40 percent to come from the world of cues and signals. And the signals that our modern world beams at us train us to want all that is "good" and nothing that is "bad." The signals do not, of course, train us to decide for ourselves what is good or bad. Instead, Big Food corporations such as Kraft, General Mills, and ConAgra spend billions of dollars— more than three billion dollars annually by Coca-Cola and Pepsico alone—to persuade us to supersize our consumption of the most fattening foods available. Meanwhile, Big Fashion spends just as much to persuade us we all should look like paper-thin supermodels. These continuous streams of competing cues— delivered through film, television, magazines, and ads for everything from cars to candy bars—encourage us to turn consumption into a compulsion that can never be satisfied. Those who fall for the commercial equation of happiness with Big Food tend to gain more weight than they need or want. Those who have a biological propensity to anorexia may instead heed the message of Big Fashion and develop a terror of fat. A third group, conditioned to believe that both Big Macs and little waistlines will bring them happiness, try to compromise by taking in more than they need—and then getting rid of it by purging, taking diet pills, or compulsively exercising. The latest and most appalling commercial trend overtly targets this last group with ads such as one for a popular Manhattan restaurant that read, "Supermodels love our pasta. It comes up as easily as it goes down."

The result of our "consuming passions" is pure profit for corporate America. McDonald's revenues alone in 2005 reached nineteen billion dollars. The U.S. diet industry takes in upwards of fifty billion dollars a year. And now Big Fitness has added a whole new layer of consumer pressure. "The models today aren't Twiggy," Brownell said, "but they're not that far from Twiggy in weight, and superimposed on that is the need to be sculpted. Thanks to a multimillion-dollar industry that runs gyms and manufactures exercise machines, there's this language—abs, delts, pecs. That pressure, of course, is unisex. I'm sure it's contributed to the rising rates of eating disorders among men. One out of every ten people with anorexia nervosa used to be male. Now that rate is one in seven."

What drives these trends is competition. If we are winners, the American Dream whispers, we will rise in status; and rising in status will make us rich, strong, lovable, and happy. "Most non-Western cultures," University of New Mexico psychologist Joel Yager told me, "give the individual very little latitude in being able to change class lines. If you're born into a low caste in India, who are you going to be? There the attitude is, don't even waste your time trying to better yourself, so rates of eating disorders are low. But in the United States, achievement, appearance, and glamour make you more marketable. Think *Pretty Woman* and *Flashdance*—the female versions of *Rocky*—coming out of nowhere and making it. The possibilities in Western culture make people more competitive—*if* they are ambitious at all. Put perfectionism into this mix, and the competitiveness becomes compulsive."

Parents who have a history of eating disorders in their families need to be especially cognizant of the cultural forces that can trigger anorexia or bulimia in perfectionistic children. An extreme emphasis on competition, achievement, and appearance—at school, within the family, or among friends—can easily lead to extreme dieting. Image-driven occupations such as modeling and acting may prove dangerous for girls who cannot accurately see or accept themselves. And athletics warrant particular attention, especially those that overtly judge performance by physical appearance. Parents need to be aware that children who are temperamentally vulnerable may be drawn to certain types of activities because they "legitimize" excessive discipline and weight loss.

It's also important to recognize, however, that all sports are not equal. Soccer, hockey, basketball, and most other team sports are by definition group efforts, so what's good for each player must also be good for the team. Or, as my son's soccer team used to yell before their games, "One for all and all for one!" If a player has anorexia, she weakens her own performance and, in her obsession, becomes emotionally alienated from her fellow players, thus becoming a liability to the team. Ideally, group sports boost precisely those critical character traits—cooperativeness, self-transcendence, and self-directedness—that protect against eating disorders. They also have a positive effect on self-esteem and confidence. All these positive effects are undermined, however, when physical appearance becomes equally or more important than performance. Nicole Bourquin, founder of the Eating Disorder Foundation of Orange

County, California, has noticed a recent rise in eating disorders among volleyball players, which directly parallels the increasing "exposure" of this sport on television. For the first time, at the 2004 Athens Olympics, beach volleyball competitors were required to wear swimsuits so skimpy that CNN commentators quipped, "Beach volleyball has now joined go-go girl dancing as perhaps the only two professions where a bikini is the required uniform." Or, as one blogger put it, echoing sentiments repeated all over the Web that summer: "It's not a sport. It's soft porn."

Sports that are specifically judged by the size and shape of an athlete's body, especially when coaches use shame as a means of "motivation," tend to breed eating disorders. Anorexia and bulimia abound in appearance events ranging from figure skating and diving to track and field and dance. The sport with the highest rate is gymnastics, which stresses not only low body weight but also a body type that is prepubescent. The problem of eating disorders in gymnastics became common knowledge after the death in 1994 of Christy Henrich. She'd begun fasting and purging after a U.S. judge at a meet in Budapest told her she'd have to lose weight if she wanted to make the Olympic team. Six years later her anorexia and bulimia led to multiple organ failure. She was twenty-two.

Henrich's death was portrayed in the press as a wake-up call to coaches and schools. Kathy Johnson and Nadia Comaneci came forward and admitted that they had had eating disorders. Cathy Rigby, a 1972 Olympian, announced that she had battled anorexia and bulimia for twelve years and had gone into cardiac arrest on two occasions as a result. The U. S. Gymnastics Federation started a hot line for athletes to call if they felt parents or coaches were pressuring them to lose weight. The Fédération Internationale de Gymnastique raised age eligibility for international competition by a year to promote a more mature body ideal. And the USA Gymnastics Athlete Wellness Program was formed to advise coaches, parents, and judges and to link them to nutritional, psychiatric, and medical specialists in eating disorders. In spite of these measures, however, a 2004 University of Oklahoma study of nearly fifteen hundred student athletes found that 42 percent of Division 1 gymnasts and cross-country runners still had disordered eating.

What makes these sports so pernicious are the official standards of appearance and control, which mirror the obsessions that drive anorexia and bulimia. Thinner is always better. Athletes must continuously compete against themselves to improve their time, form, or routine. No achievement is ever good enough, and there is no clear dividing line between passion and compulsion. Given the hours of practice and dedication required to win, it's assumed that a certain amount of compulsiveness is actually necessary. No one ever questions winning as the ultimate goal.

Even in a looks-fixated sport like gymnastics, however, Kelly Brownell believes it's essential to draw a distinction between the girl who takes up the balance beam because it makes her feel like she's walking on air and the girl who walks the beam as a means of self-punishment. Those who are naturally prone to anorexia or bulimia, Brownell said, "have the right traits to be competitive—they're very hard workers, they can control their eating and their weight." By nature, they tend to become as compulsive about their sport as they are about dieting. They also tend to burn out or injure themselves from overtraining, and perhaps most important of all, they derive little or no joy from their grueling dedication. "But there's another group," he continued, "who are drawn to the sport for the sport's sake," who subscribe to the dictionary definition of sport as "activity that gives enjoyment or recreation." These athletes compete out of genuine passion for their particular event.

This passionate group may also develop an eating disorder in the push to make weight, but Brownell's research has shown that they tend to recover quickly once the pressure is off. He told me about a study he had done with college wrestlers who were required to drop weight in order to compete. The way they fasted, binged, purged, and exercised during the season did meet the technical criteria for anorexia and bulimia. "But when the off season came, they'd be back to their normal selves again." Similar studies have found that the competitors who have long-term problems with eating disorders tend to be those whose temperaments predisposed them to these disorders before they entered their sport. The majority of athletes, even in gymnastics, resume normal eating as soon as they retire. What's more, most credit their athletic careers with raising their self-esteem and self-confidence—exactly the opposite effect usually associated with eating disorders. This doesn't diminish the physical dangers of sport-induced eating disorders, but it does suggest that the answer may be to reevaluate the emphasis on weight within the sports world and pay more attention to the mental as well as physical health of competitors—and not just condemn the sports outright.

Exercise is a natural and necessary component of life. It is essential for health. And while it can ignite eating disorders, it can also cure them. As Jean Bristol explained it to me, the key is motivation.

When Jean first e-mailed me, describing the passion that had cured her bulimia as a "wild ride," I thought she was being dramatic. I learned through our subsequent correspondence that the phrase was both literal and an understatement. The broad strokes of Jean's life read like elements of a *Vanity Fair* feature. After graduating from Cornell, she married a young industrialist from one of Argentina's most prominent families. He bred horses and ran television networks. Jean was a painter. Over their fifteen years together, they lived in Brazil, Paraguay, and Chile. They had two sons, full-time servants, and several stables of Thoroughbreds that they both loved to ride. But Jean's husband wanted her to be a socialite wife and stay-at-home mother. She was starting to show her work at galleries and was not about to quit her art. Now they were separated, and Jean feared her husband was going to demand custody of her little boys. I was surprised, then, by Jean's upbeat attitude when she returned to the States from Buenos Aires to visit her family in Virginia and we finally spoke by phone. "One of the reasons we're getting divorced," she said, "is that he's a person who needs and needs to be needed. I'm very independent. That's why the bulimia was so weird. I'm so darn secure with myself."

Such declarations always seem to me suspect, and Jean was right that her history of bulimia belied her supposed security. But as we talked she admitted she hadn't always been so self-assured. Like many girls who develop bulimia, she'd grown up with two warring emotional tendencies—to withdraw shyly into herself and to turn pugnacious whenever she felt threatened. She had no clear ambitions or desires. The one unifying force in her life, though she didn't realize it until her twenties, was her connection to horses.

Jean's mother raises and shows saddlebred horses. Jean began showing at nine. She always loved the horses, but the show world often focused less on the animals than on how riders looked on the horse, their competitive ranking on the show circuit, and their status in show horse society. The terrible paradox is that while horses are now becoming recognized as a therapeutic ally in treating eating disorders, certain events within the world of equestrian competition make it as prime a breeding ground as gymnastics for anorexia and bulimia. Equitation, in which the rider's performance and control are judged as important or more important than the performance of the horse, especially seems to promote disordered eating. In his book *Hunter Seat Equitation*, master equestrian George Morris wrote, "Rarely can someone be too thin for this sport." And in 2005, U.S. Equestrian Federation judge Andrea Meek acknowledged in *Horse Illustrated* that thin riders usually place above heavier riders in equitation, not because of any difference in ability but because they have a cleaner line and she, after all, was "judging the overall look of the horse and rider."

"I knew a lot of people who were anorexic," Jean told me of the world in which she was raised. "Owners and trainers."

Jean escaped this pressure as a child because she was naturally small and slim and loved all forms of exercise. But at seventeen while visiting Spain as a high school exchange student she injured her ankle. The resulting inactivity—plus the paella, flan, and churros her Spanish family lavished on her—caused her to gain ten pounds in two months. Jean panicked when the scale registered 115. (Though she wasn't consciously aware of it at the time, this number carries particular significance in the horse world because it is the upper weight limit for professional jockeys. To "help" jockeys stay below this limit, track locker rooms are actually equipped with step machines *inside* saunas, basins specifically designed for vomiting, and ready supplies of diet pills and diuretics.) Jean felt compelled to lose every ounce she'd gained, by whatever means worked fastest. By the time she returned to the States to begin her freshman year of college, purging had become part of her daily routine. By sophomore year she was taking in and rejecting food the same way she did beer, work, and boyfriends. "Whatever I do," she told me, "I throw myself into it . . . and I'll forget it just as quickly afterward. There is this impulse to try the limits."

One of Jean's impulses was to return to Spain to pursue a romance with a man she'd met there. She arranged to spend her junior year in Madrid. But she quickly reached the limit of her interest in the young man, and what came next was an "existential crisis. It all started early one morning, when I got to campus, took one look at the Political Science Building and got back on the bus. I returned to Madrid, walked into El Corte Ingles department store, with every intention of buying Milan Kundera's *Incredible Lightness of Being*. I found it easily on the shelf, stuck it under my arm—I had no purse or bag, not even a jacket—and walked out of the store. I walked all over Madrid until late that night. For weeks I stole chocolate, food, and drink and gave it to the bums on the street. I walked out of another department store with a wool blanket slung around my shoulders, walked straight across the street to where a homeless man slept in the same doorway, and I gave him the blanket. I didn't go to class. I just kind of went nuts for a while."

The only thing Jean knew for sure was that she missed horses and riding. The riding clubs in Madrid cost more than she could afford, so a friend suggested she go to the track. In Spain, trainers welcomed volunteers to exercise their horses—it saved them the cost of professional gallopers. Jean was five foot two and by then weighed 105. "I just walked in and said I was looking for a horse to ride, and they said, 'Here.'" One potential problem was that she had never ridden a racehorse. She was used to trotting and jumping under show conditions, riding that was about being seen and controlled, not releasing the horse's full power. Her first time around the track at speed, Jean felt exhilarated. She signed on to ride every day, and soon her appetite for galloping became insatiable. This new and authentic passion eliminated her compulsion to purge almost overnight.

"What changed?" I asked.

"It's a focus thing. It gets you away from the demons that are wandering around in your head. If you're totally focused on what you're doing, you're not thinking sixty million circles around whatever you think you should be. It's getting comfortable with yourself. And the whole thing with eating disorders is being comfortable with who you are." Galloping, she found, was as liberating as equitation was constrained, as real as showing could be superficial. "My younger brother talks about martial arts as the idea of feeling at one with yourself and yet transcending yourself, having instantaneous perception and reaction to your environment. That happened to me riding horses. If you persist long enough you learn everything very quickly and everything happens automatically, and you don't have this delay between present and past. You're all in the present."

What Jean was describing, it seemed to me, was a state that some might call the essence of passion. Social psychologist

Mihaly Csikszentmihalyi calls it "flow." When you're in this state, you're fully engaged and focused in an activity that you love, that's well matched to your personal skills, and that gives you a sense of control; this activity causes you to lose awareness of time and yourself even as you feel more connected to the larger world or life around you; and the experience itself feels like a reward, regardless of the end result of your efforts. Csikszentmihalyi found that research subjects could reach this altered state through activities as cerebral as prayer and meditation; as creative as writing or painting; or as physical as yoga, gymnastics, or riding. The state itself, he wrote in *Flow: The Psychology of Optimal Experience*, was characterized by "a sense of discovery, a creative feeling of transporting the person into a new reality. It pushed the person to higher levels of performance, and led to previously undreamed-of states of consciousness. In short, it transformed the self by making it more complex."

"I have been known to say I rowed my way out of anorexia," Caroline Knapp wrote of her utter captivation with a sport that she compared to aquatic tightrope walking. Like galloping a racehorse, sculling requires nerve, intense concentration, physical effort, and mastery. When rowing, Knapp recalled, "I began to feel something I may never quite have felt as a woman before, which was integrated and strong and whole, the body as a piece, the body as responsive and connected to the mind, the body as a worthy place to live." What Knapp discovered as she sculled and Jean realized as she galloped was that the ultimate experience of control is achieved, paradoxically, when we are least worried about control. The rider arrives as if by magic at the finish line, the writer at the end of a chapter, the dancer at her final pirouette.

This state can also be reached through study, but, again, the key is to let go of *intention* and allow the complete, relaxed flow of *attention*. Karen Armstrong wrote of the shift that she experienced in reading as she attained this state: "Insight does not always come to order, and there will certainly be no renaissance if you are merely trying to 'get' something for yourself. As soon as I stopped trying to exploit my literary skills to advance my career or enhance my reputation, I found that I was opening myself to the text, could lose myself in the beauty of the words and in the wisdom of the writer. It was a kind of *ekstasis* . . . a going beyond the self."

What *must* happen or what *should* happen occurs naturally when we fully attend to what *is* happening. This is the exact opposite of compulsive competition. "You can't be carrying around baggage or problems," Jean Bristol reflected. "You have to set it aside, empty your mind of all that stuff, so it drives you out of yourself and into the moment." And "the moment" is the life that we are living right now—"every moment afresh," as Virginia Woolf wrote in *Mrs. Dalloway*. It is our choice, and our choice alone, whether to make the most of this moment or the least, whether to live it out of passion or out of fear.

The sad reality is that so many choose to let their compulsions consume their lives. Jean was in the distinct minority of women I interviewed who had learned this lesson before her thirtieth birthday. The good news is that for many of the others, the best moments of their lives had come with age.

11

THE WISDOM OF AGE
Maturity in a Youth Culture

> The compensation of growing old . . . was
> simply this; that the passions remain as strong as
> ever, but one has gained—at last!—the power
> which adds the supreme flavour to existence,—
> the power of taking hold of experience, of turn-
> ing it round, slowly, in the light.
> —Virginia Woolf, *Mrs. Dalloway*

THERE WAS SUCH FEEDBACK for not feeding yourself." This was
how Vanessa Quintero recalled her free fall into anorexia nervosa
in her late forties. The perfectionist I'd first met preparing for her
book group with edible pansies and silver arranged in military
formation might, however, have been talking about American
women and girls of any age or weight. There is no question that
females in this culture are encouraged and rewarded when they
physically make less of themselves. As study after study has
shown, they begin to absorb this message in elementary school,
begin acting on it by middle school, and too often become sick
with it by high school. But Vanessa's story illustrates that the
damage doesn't always stop, or even slow down, there.

The evening I returned to her home to interview her, Vanessa welcomed me with the same impeccable hospitality she'd shown at our first meeting. The coffee table was set with bone china, silver plates piled with homemade bitter fudge, and individual teapots dosed with imported green tea in fabric sacks. Vanessa sat on the edge of her chair, flanked by side tables arranged with silver-framed photographs of her and John, her husband of thirty years, and their now grown son, Ben. She held her cup and saucer as if entertaining Nancy Reagan.

"Where is Ben now?" I asked to break the tension.

Vanessa beamed. "He's in a wonderful community in New Mexico."

"Community?"

"Ben is autistic." I took a closer look at Ben's photographs. He resembled the actor Fred Gwynne, except that his gaze didn't quite connect with the camera. Vanessa smiled at the picture. "He can't live on his own, but he knows every musical ever recorded. He can sing the show tunes by heart. I think it's in his blood. John's mother was an actress and singer." She motioned to a picture on the wall of a robust Jane Russell look-alike circa 1960. Vanessa's tone shifted as perceptibly as a changed CD. "Speaking of people with eating disorders."

John's mother, Vanessa told me, was truly a larger-than-life character. "Brilliant, talented, intelligent, and completely self-absorbed. She blamed her son for losing her figure and her career. She was totally irresponsible—the exact opposite of me." Vanessa ascribed a highly specific meaning to the word *irresponsible*, at least when it came to fat and figures. Her own mother weighed 236 pounds. Her sister weighed 200. Her father had died from complications of obesity in his sixties. "His watchword was 'A little bit won't hurt you.' My mother-in-law's was 'You want to eat a whole cake, get a fork.' She struggled and suffered her entire life with weight. She had a sister with a perfect body, but she was always chubby. Her father ridiculed her. She said she'd rather die than be fat. That's exactly what happened."

I looked again at the Rubenesque face in the picture. "*What exactly happened?*"

Vanessa explained that her mother-in-law had been one of the first people in New York to have gastric bypass surgery, which at the time consisted of separating the small intestine from the large intestine, so food went directly into the bowel, eliminating about 85 percent of nutrients. The procedure was designed as a drastic and temporary measure to reduce weight in the morbidly obese. Patients had to take massive supplements and were closely monitored. When they reached their target weight, the intestines were reattached and the patient was expected to follow a maintenance diet. Vanessa's mother-in-law lost fifty pounds before the reattachment. "But she gained it all right back. She had no proper health habits. She had the surgery again, without telling any of us, and refused to be hooked up again. She ducked her doctors. Her body was severely malnourished. Her kidneys began to fail. We found out because she wanted a kidney transplant from my husband, but there was no time." Vanessa glared at the photograph. "Even on her deathbed she swore she wouldn't be hooked back up again. She wanted a quick fix. Painless."

I didn't know what to say. The horror of this story was almost beyond imagining, but Vanessa clearly wasn't asking for sympathy.

"I'm very judgmental," she admitted, waving a hand at her mother-in-law as if to say, Over, done with. "I don't judge people by their car or their jewelry or their home. But I do judge them by the way they receive the world and the way they want to be responsible. I like responsible, organized, caring, kind people. So when I see people doing things that are out of whack, it seems self-indulgent. If I see an overweight person drinking a big Coke and eating hamburgers and fries, I want to say, 'Your arteries! Have you thought about your arteries?' I want to be like a prophet. 'Listen up, group! The reason you're fat is that you're eating crap!'"

"And this goes back to your childhood, growing up with overweight parents?"

Vanessa was animated now and vexed. "I have a zealot's personality. I've always been concerned about food. Not to lose weight but to take responsibility for my health by the kind of food I ate. I felt I could control it. I would call it a healthy predisposition for understanding food, reading the labels, and knowing how many vitamins are in celery as opposed to carrots, and fat grams. I always had this interest."

Curiously, Vanessa seemed to have reversed the typical course of eating disorders, which begins with self-destructive obsession with food and gradually tapers into more health-conscious regimens. I asked, "When and how did you shift into anorexia?"

"It started when I was forty-five. I had a blood test, and my blood sugar was out of range. I wasn't heavy, but my father and his family all had diabetes. So I went to a nutritionist, and she put me on a diabetic diet and said, 'The best thing for you is exercise.' Well, that's all she needed to say. I got a personal trainer. I wanted to please him and show him that a forty-five-year-old woman could beat a twenty-five-year-old man in sit-ups. Being strong was so exhilarating, and not eating enough made me feel very high and in control and powerful and young. And racy and beautiful. Wow, to get into size three Gap jeans at this age! I became obsessive about the scale. I put it by my bed. I would weigh myself in the morning, the evening, whenever I had a spare moment. I would be elated if it went down a couple of points. If it went up, I went, What have I done, what have I eaten, this is out of control!"

"What did your husband say?"

She blinked. "You know, I don't remember."

"He didn't say your behavior was odd? He didn't think you were losing too much weight?"

"He's in the back. Shall we ask him?" But Vanessa didn't wait for my answer. I'd piqued her curiosity.

John came in, a large unassuming man in a dark Hawaiian shirt, and dropped into an armchair opposite his wife. Vanessa's question seemed to catch him off guard. "I never considered you anorexic," he said. "You were real buff, and whatever else kicks in before the changes you go through . . . you were just very petite."

At her low point, Vanessa weighed 103 pounds—a weight I'd guess to be slightly less than half of John's as he sat before me. Together with the hours she'd spent at the gym, the number of times she weighed herself each day, the amount of energy she'd poured into slicing her portions and assessing her reflection, this weight qualified her, in medical terms, for "subclinical anorexia nervosa"—not ill enough to require hospitalization, but dangerously close.

"Remember the chart I kept?" Vanessa prodded him. "What did you think about my losing all that weight?"

He folded his arms across his chest. "You were never too thin. I've seen people where you see bones."

"I was taking good habits to an extreme."

"You just were consistent. You didn't deviate."

I wondered how much more consistent Vanessa would have had to be before her husband noticed that, in her own terms, she was doing something out of whack. But I was concerned that if this went on any longer John's remarks just might push Vanessa to prove her "fantastic" compulsiveness with a relapse. I thanked him for his perspective, and he returned to his study.

Vanessa fussed with her bangs for a minute after he'd gone. Then she brightened. "John is a dear. He thinks it's my nature to be overly concerned about what I can control."

I conceded that I'd noticed the same thing. "But I think one reason eating disorders happen is that so often nobody notices there's a problem until it's serious. One woman told me her mother said she looked great when she weighed eighty-eight pounds."

"People *would* say wonderful things," Vanessa said a little wistfully. "'Oh, what self-discipline! How can you deny yourself these things! My gosh, the willpower!'"

"I always wonder why we applaud women for denying themselves."

Vanessa seemed not to hear me. "I thought, hmm, people think I'm wonderful, when I'm just really taking charge of my life."

"What else was going on in your life at the time?"

She had to stop and think. This was ten years ago now. Ben had been about nineteen, six feet tall, out of school, but unable to live independently. Vanessa and John had moved him into a residential care program shortly before Vanessa began working out with her trainer. It was the first time she had been separated from her son, and she wasn't sure about the program, from which they would, in fact, later move him to his current community. Meanwhile, John was facing a possible layoff at his engineering firm, and Vanessa had just been promoted as head of personnel at her publishing company.

"A lot of changes hitting you at once," I said. "A lot of shifting roles. Not easy for somebody who needs to have everything under control."

Vanessa smiled graciously at my ribbing. "I have a psychologist friend who told me, 'You have an anorexic personality.' I wanted to say, No, I'm healthy! I'm healthy and proud of it. But that's when I knew I'd overdone it. I'd lost my personal relationship with food, and society was controlling it and me. I didn't want to be like that, but once I stopped what would happen? Would I balloon up? Anxiety kicked in."

I asked what had finally turned her around.

"My hair started falling out. I was in the shower, and I would look, and there was more and more. I panicked. My body decided to be more powerful than my mind, and I decided to stop fighting it."

And then there was menopause. "That was definitely part of the obsession, the dread of menopause, but once it happened I realized, this is okay. I can be a partner with nature instead of trying to control it." By this time Vanessa was fifty. Her periods had lapsed. Her temperature rose and fell as if some invisible prankster had seized her body's thermometer—a phenomenon so weird it was almost as fascinating as it was infuriating. And regardless of her weight, the substance of her body seemed to be thickening, softening, and slowing. Her thighs grew proportionally thinner, her waist thicker as hormonal changes redistributed her body fat. It reminded her of adolescence, when her physiological terrain seemed to shift between homeroom and lunch. As a teenager Vanessa had been too busy taking care of her family—her little sister, her father in the hospital when he became ill, her severely depressed mother—to pay much attention to her developing body except to vow to herself that she would never become overweight like her parents. And she never had. She reminded herself of this as she stopped trying to force her body into unnatural dimensions at midlife.

"Enough was enough. I decided to be the best-looking person I could be, but *for my age*—a healthy and mature woman, hips and all. I wasn't going to be fat, but I didn't want to be a teenager, either. I wanted a different type of power."

I asked what she meant by power.

"I was an object during the real heavy control and exercise obsession. Now I want to be a person." She toasted me with her teacup. "Who am I living for? Myself or society?"

Vanessa leaned forward, the zealot unleashed with a new urgency. "If somebody said, 'You can gain five pounds all over your body and live healthily until you're eighty-nine,' I would do it in a heartbeat."

By all rational, objective standards, it's hard to imagine anyone turning down a promise of longevity just because it came with a few extra pounds. But most women in our culture are not conditioned by rational, objective standards. More than 70 percent of normal-weight women over thirty are dissatisfied with their weight. In a large nationwide poll conducted in 1997, an astonishing 39 percent of normal-weight women said they would willingly *die* three years early if it meant they could reach their desired weight now. Fifteen percent would have traded as much as five years of life for a thinner body. On average, these women stood five feet five inches tall and weighed 140, so they would have cut their lives short to lose just fifteen pounds. Whether or not they had diagnosable eating disorders, these women's level of desperation and self-loathing indicate a serious problem not just individually but societally. A large part of this problem is the double standard that our society applies to beauty and aging.

While almost every culture treats beauty as a woman's default currency, the tragedy in our Western world is that beauty has been reduced to two narrow standards, youthfulness and thinness, which implicitly exclude women as they age. So while men become distinguished, handsome, elegant, silver haired, and stately—especially if they are wealthy—even the richest, most elegant women are said to "lose their looks" as soon as their hair starts to gray. Crow's-feet, laugh lines, spreading midriffs, and age spots are unisex phenomena, but these phrases are used almost exclusively and negatively by and about women. That's because only women experience these signals of age as a threat to their social, sexual, and professional status. As an actress friend in her early forties said to me, "I walk down the street and men look past me as if I'm invisible."

Kathryn Zerbe, professor of psychiatry at Oregon Health & Science University, believes that midlife eating disorders represent a desperate attempt to deny these losses. We resent losing our youth, she says. We regret our mistakes. We deny that we no longer have the stamina for careers that have yet to peak, and above all, we cannot face the fact that we are running out of time. But if we fixate on our weight we don't have to think about what really frightens us.

I am now in my early fifties, so I know these losses firsthand.

Physical pain and frailty shadow family reunions. My parents have turned elderly. And I can feel myself losing the sense of limitless possibility that alternately vexed and reassured my younger mind. I have lost the hope of bearing any future children, and, most confusing of all, I have lost to adulthood the children who once were my babies. Make no mistake, my son and stepson today are interesting, kind, active individuals leading their own productive lives, and they do me proud. But the way they smelled as little boys, the way they held my hand, the way they pounded in and out of the house and needed me to soothe or referee their hurt feelings—all of that is no more. My maternal job has been downsized to the role of occasional driver, cook, editor, and cheerleader; and my looks have become a lined and sagging metaphor for the powerlessness I feel in the face of youth's vitality. My once children are gaining on me, while increasing numbers of my peers are divorced or widowed or gone. I recognize that to dwell on loss is to ignore the gains that come only with age. I have survived my years of self-denial and the crucible of separation. My marriage is sweeter than ever, my sons are thriving, and my days are full of purpose and passion. Still, the gains do not render the losses less real. They deserve to be respected, not denied.

Whether eating disorders occur in adolescence or middle age, denial *is* both their essential ingredient and their function. Adolescents are buffeted by tumultuous physical, social, and emotional change as they lose their youth and are forced toward a new level of maturity. So are middle-aged women. Both teen and midlife anorexics complain they don't feel seen or known, while bulimics young and older typically feel ashamed of how they're seen. Grown women with vulnerable temperaments, in other words, resort to eating disorders for all the same reasons that girls do. At establishments like the Renfrew Center, women over thirty now make up a full third of residential eating disorder patients. Every therapist I interviewed in the course of writing this book was seeing older anorexic and bulimic patients. One patient had begun restricting food in her fifties after losing her only child. Dieting distracted the woman from her grief, which she refused to discuss. Eventually her husband left her. He remarried and started another family. She couldn't talk about that loss, either. Instead she kept on losing weight until she was finally referred for treatment.

Sometimes, it seems as if the only people who do recognize the losses of aging women are those who exploit them. Cosmetics companies, fitness gurus, and plastic surgeons all promote the grand illusion, guaranteed to let their customers down, that if we spend, sacrifice, and try hard enough to acquire a youthful face and body we can reverse or neutralize the harder realities of age. Women prone to eating disorders make easy prey for these peddlers of imitation youth. I live in Los Angeles, perhaps the world's capital of plastic surgery; and while it's easy to make jokes about celebrity breast implants, crooked eye lifts, and botched Botox treatments, what I see when I stroll the streets of Beverly Hills are legions of sad, brittle elderly women who no longer look quite human. With their cheeks pulled up to their foreheads, their shrunken bodies, inflated lips and breasts, and hair dyed to a crisp, they attract stares that may make them feel visible, but those same younger men and women who stare then turn and roll their eyes. These women's drastic attempts to deny the reality of age turn them into objects of pity. What I find particularly sad is the joylessness in these women's faces. Despite their painful, expensive, and time-devouring efforts to turn back the biological clock, their expressions remind me of my own reflection during my anorexic years—a clench of intense, if denied, anxiety. Eating disorders are so common among women seeking cosmetic surgery that therapists now advise plastic surgeons to routinely screen for anorexia and bulimia. Sadly, cosmetic surgery rates jumped 24 percent between 2000 and 2005, 5 percent in 2004 alone.

"We are what we are devoted to," Erich Fromm wrote, "and what we are devoted to is what motivates our conduct." As I began writing this chapter, relief efforts were under way following Hurricane Katrina. In Louisiana, Alabama, and Mississippi, thousands of volunteers were devoting themselves to helping feed and house those left homeless by the disaster. On the other side of the world, my friend Deborah, fifty-three, recently divorced, and in the middle of a career change from Hollywood screenwriting to international conflict resolution, was devoting her summer to helping Liberian refugees establish schools for their children in Guinea. Other middle-aged women I know have chosen to adopt children or launch new careers in the arts. I went back to school for a master's degree that would equip me to teach. These are all examples of what Erik Erikson calls *generativity:* "the concern for establishing and guiding the next generation." By this he did not mean only caring for one's own children but all forms of altruistic concern and creativity that are sustained by love. Erikson, writing a decade before Fromm, declared, "We are what we love."

The distinction between *devotion* and *love* is critical. Some of us are plenty capable of devoting ourselves to fitting into a size 2, getting our eyes or breasts "fixed," or tucking in several hours a day on the StairMaster in hopes of reversing our beauty clock. But it's hard to imagine love playing any part in such devotions. "Love," Erikson wrote, "binds into a 'way of life' the affiliations of competition and co-operation, production and procreation." In other words, love builds character. It makes us distinctive yet balanced individuals. And it gains us strength and maturity. When we feel bored, empty, or envious of others just for enjoying life, it's a sign that love is missing or has failed us. And without love, Erikson wrote, we tend to regress to the habits, illusions, and pathologies of our lost youth.

Love fails us in a host of ways. When I was twenty I thought midlife divorces were a cliché. By the time I was forty I saw this cliché playing out in half the households of my son's elementary school classmates. Eventually, it would threaten our own, and I came to understand that the cliché was based on the most fundamental of all human fears. Men and women both have a tendency to panic at the first strong whiff of their own mortality, whether it comes in the form of a fortieth birthday, a heart attack, a layoff or demotion at work, or an unsettling shift in libido. Devoted fathers start complaining about having "only one life." Conventional men talk longingly of "adventures." Women, in my experience, tend to respond to such talk with an equal and opposite reaction. They cry. They accuse. They have affairs. They go to the gym. They shop for black and red lingerie at Victoria's Secret. They struggle to look as young as their husbands are acting, perhaps as young as the women their husbands are secretly seeing. And if they've ever had an eating disorder, they may well relapse now. One former anorexic I know, a news photographer whose stock-in-trade is objectivity, told herself after she was separated that she'd never looked better. She had a friend take a picture of her on the beach and sent it to her husband. She wanted to show him how brilliantly she was faring without him. She hoped to arouse his jealousy. Instead he called to ask if she was sick. She looked so skeletally thin he advised her to see a doctor.

"That's the real illness in most mental illness," Sally said. "You're so unhappy with yourself, you're either running away from it or punishing yourself or obsessing."

Sally Malloy has been my friend for almost twenty years. Our sons went to preschool together. She is a pediatrician who specializes in treating children with learning disorders. Both she and her sister have histories of eating disorders. When she learned I was writing this book she offered to tell her story of the "epiphany" she'd experienced at forty-eight.

"I used to be the impulsive child who tried to please and always moved too fast, broke something, said the wrong thing, was irritating." As Sally talked, very fast, with an intensity that made me hope my tape recorder functioned properly because I couldn't possibly keep up with her in my notebook, I had no difficulty picturing her as a quicksilver child. The way she sat cross-legged in her garden wearing green cords and a white T-shirt, barefoot; no makeup; her long, dark mane of hair loose around her shoulders, she might still have been fifteen. Sally was bulimic for seven years—from age fifteen to twenty-two, bingeing and purging up to five times a day. Her younger sister Nora, was anorexic, beginning in high school when she dropped to 70 pounds. Their parents, an engineer father and homemaker mother, had been upstanding members of their suburban Illinois community, so concerned about what the neighbors would think that they refused even to consider sending Nora to a psychologist.

With Sally's support her sister cycled out of anorexia but then moved on to drugs and alcohol, suffered from chronic depression, and only began to feel normal and healthy after she met her partner, Trudi, and came out sexually in her early thirties. "Nora suffered much, much worse than I ever did," Sally told me. But Sally's own eating disorder also went undiagnosed and untreated. Although she stopped vomiting on her own, she admitted, "I still had a very bulimic way of seeing the world. Very much holding on to things and wanting to succeed. Success being tied to labels and things, without really understanding. Just sort of chasing but not knowing what I was chasing." She'd replaced bulimia first with smoking, then work, "driving to achieve a name, fame, as a means of control, of proving I deserved some attention."

I had observed this in Sally, without putting it in those terms. In the years I'd known her she had "binged and purged" on kickboxing, marathon running, Rollerblading, spinning, Pilates, foreign vacations, home decorating and entertaining, as well as professional megaprojects, and, on occasion, friends. Her enthusiasms tended to be intense, compulsive, short-lived, and often strangely at odds with Sally's nature. This is one of the smartest women I know. She freely admits she's a terrible cook and a bit of a klutz, has no real fashion sense, and knows only what her decorator tells her about home design; but she rises at five every morning to work on lectures, grant proposals, and scientific papers before getting her three kids up and off to school, and then spends her days with patients, the families in her research projects, and students. Her three children and her husband, Jay, who's been with her since they were seventeen, are the constants in Sally's life. Yet she typically would stopper her professional persona around her family. When my husband and I went out to dinner with Sally and Jay, she would point her conversation to the kids' latest escapades or Jay's latest entrepreneurial ventures. Admittedly, Jay's accomplishments are impressive. One of five siblings who never went to college, he catapulted himself from blue-collar beginnings to a net worth of many millions. And although he was an active alcoholic during the same years when Sally was bulimic, he's been sober now for nearly thirty years. But Sally's deference to her husband always seemed as cautious as it was respectful. I often had the sense that she was holding herself back and that the need for release was what drove her binges in work, exercise, spending, traveling, social networking—all of which left her still hungry.

Then, at forty-seven, she discovered a small freckle on her arm that turned out to be in situ melanoma. "The thought of death overwhelmed me. My father had just died. My mother, a nonsmoker all her life, had recently been diagnosed with lung cancer. Now the life I thought I loved so much, the children, the husband, the house, my possessions, were to be taken from me, too. I thought I wouldn't live to fifty." Sally's panic escalated until, one morning as she was racing to get the kids to school, "a bizarre crystal light emerges in my left visual field. I blink. It doesn't go away. I blink again. It's not disappearing. My mind races to the only rational conclusion—metastasized cancer to the brain; neurological impairment; death is imminent." Sally's medical knowledge served only to convince her she was doomed. Neither her oncologist nor her psychiatrist could reassure her. Desperate for some dramatic change that would restore her sense of control, she took a leave of absence from work and turned to alternative medicine, yoga, massage. Never before religious, she began practicing Zen meditation an hour or two each day. She adopted a Buddhist vegetarian diet and read voraciously about mindfulness and its effect on brain chemistry. She expanded her circle of friends through her yoga and meditation centers. Now she's grateful.

"I had a great awakening that I was going to die. That reality that's right in front of you, that you could die today—it became so real that I could either shut down and move away from it or I could go into it and say, of course, I'm going to die and that *is* life. Suddenly I realized the chase for fame and fortune is all based on fear and avoidance of death. I felt the beauty of life as it is, each moment as it arises. Everywhere I turned, I saw this beauty—spiderwebs, wrinkled bedsheets, the light in the morning, and people of all shapes and sizes. I lost that perspective of viewing the world through judgmental eyes—too big, too small—and just saw things as they were. When you get into this open-minded space, you have all the time in the world because in every moment is all the time you have. So I no longer hurry. I'm not rushing people anymore, and I'm much more comfortable with things as they are."

Sally described the "epiphany" as a massive reorganization of her worldview. "It happened over a really short period of time—thirty, forty days. It was enlightenment, if you want to know. I was in an extremely surreal state of feeling extremely connected. I know a lot about mania and hypomania, and I believe that when people are going into a hypomania, they're often experiencing what I experienced. Remember, I was an atheist. I don't believe in a monotheistic god. I don't have any religious belief system, and I don't believe in organized religion. I truly believe it's all about inner discovery and finding the deep understanding of our interconnectedness in the sense that whatever has happened to you is as if it's happened to me. You become so interconnected with other people that you barely draw a distinction between another and yourself. Which means that you become incredibly compassionate, and it shifts the way you act in the world."

She compared the effect to giving birth and bonding with one's newborn child. "That sense of self-transcendence. So much of the aftermath of the epiphany is like that—I love myself. I know myself. I care about myself. Therefore I can truly know and love other people."

Sally's passion for mindfulness and meditation seemed substantial and enduring, but I wondered how she felt her new regimen had changed her "bulimic way of seeing the world."

"Your world is so much your mind and what you create." She cupped her hands to either side of her face, like blinders, then pulled them away. "In the past I was always very judgmental; I'm still judgmental—the human side of me—but now if I say something with a judgmental tone, my kids will immediately say, 'Mom! It's that judgmental thing.' And I can see it now, where before I'd have been too into denial. It's all so funny that you can get so caught up in stuff. So I laugh a lot. I always did, but now I *really* laugh a lot. I became a painter, did you know? I have a whole art studio. I paint three hours a day. Painting and writing. The creativity is unbelievable, and I don't feel the pressure for time anymore."

Sally looked at her watch and unfolded herself. She had an appointment to have her hair colored.

I lifted an eyebrow, and she laughed. "I do still dye my hair and I work out and am careful what I eat, but I color my hair in a salon that's become sort of a family to me—I spend my time talking with each person there. And working out is a kind of active meditation, and when I eat and drink I think about where the food came from and pay attention to how it will sustain my body. Everything is interconnected."

Mounting scientific evidence shows that mindfulness— gained through practices such as meditation, yoga, deep breathing, and tai chi—changes the brain for the better. University of Wisconsin researchers have found that Tibetan monks skilled in meditation have high levels of activity to the far left of the prefrontal cortex—a region of the brain associated with compassion, contentment, and calm. The same researchers found that people who are highly stressed, angry, depressed, and anxious show a pattern of persistent activity in the *right* prefrontal cortex, the area that commands hypervigilance. They found that stress also tends to lower the resilience of the immune system. The Wisconsin data suggest that people are born with a set point for mood just as they are born with a set point for weight—a general range that constitutes their personal norm. People who dread death and believe the world is coming to an end tend to show more consistent activity farther to the right of the brain than do people who can't wait to see what each day has in store for them. This may help to explain why some people sail into old age while others crumble under the weight of normal midlife losses. But the example of the Tibetan monks prompted Richard Davidson, the neuroscientist who leads the Wisconsin research, to wonder if meditation could be used intentionally to shift that set point to the left. He tested the question on two groups of stressed-out volunteers who were given flu shots. One group was also given training in meditation. After just eight weeks, only the meditating group's brain activity had shifted measurably toward the left, "happy" side of the prefrontal cortex. These same volunteers reported feeling more engaged in their work, more energized, and less anxious. They also had improved immune response to the flu shot.

There was more to Sally's conversion, however, than personal bliss. The components of Sally's new mindfulness matched the traits of character. Meditation involved *self-transcendence*—spirituality, faith, and an experience of being connected through one's senses with a universe much larger than one's own body. What Sally was now *doing* with her mindfulness—engaging other like-minded colleagues in building a center to teach and study the benefits of meditation—was a form of *cooperativeness*. These were human connections Sally was forming, not for her own benefit but to explore ideas that might help others. While she might have some self-interest in seeing her ideas borne out, Sally's only financial interest in this project was as a donor. Nor was she doing it for the credit; her university would absorb that. Her *self-directed* desire was simply to explore and expand her vision.

Sally's basic temperament hadn't changed and didn't need to. She still was impulsive, quick minded, and curious, still eager to please and wary of upsetting her husband and kids. She still had a powerful drive to succeed. But now she was paying more attention to the ways she channeled that drive, and she was more concerned with reaching out to people than judging or being judged by them. Success had taken on new and varied meanings as she learned to satisfy appetites that she only now, in her fifties, could fully appreciate.

One of the appetites many of us cultivate as we grow older is, oddly enough, for beauty. I say oddly because beauty is so insistently linked with youth that it seems at times as if no one over thirty—especially a "mature" woman—should even breathe the word. But that definition of beauty is the one our culture drills into us. It's that sly, seductive, sex-infused beauty that teenagers strive so to imitate. As we get older and our hormones calm down, there's no reason we *should* define beauty by the standards of adolescents. As Sally had discovered, we are free to explore beauty of a kind much larger, more powerful, and more moving than could ever be captured in a fashion photograph. I can best illustrate what I mean by describing some of the images that have prompted me to take photographs in this, my fifty-second year: a line of green figs, round and full as breasts; two reflected trees reaching across a pond, their topmost branches touching as sweetly as Adam touching God on the ceiling of the Sistine Chapel; the landscape of Vermont looking brown and moist and painterly during a freak warm snap in January; a rose in close-up, pale peach petals spiraling outward with the mathematical precision of a nautilus; snow enveloping clapboard houses, draping the lawns around them in white, and rendering time as irrelevant as a clock turned back to 1912.

Or I can tell you this story, which has stayed with me for more than ten years now. I don't recall the name of the man being interviewed, but I do recall that he was an Italian Holocaust survivor, in his seventies at the time of the radio broadcast. Not a fabulously wealthy or a particularly handsome man, he nevertheless took tremendous joy in the art of clothing. He invested carefully in his suits, often having them made by tailors who had become his personal friends. He brought silks of unusual colors back from his business trips abroad and had them made into ties and shirts with equally unusual detailing. He paid attention to texture and pattern and wore his clothes with a flair that had nothing to do with the size or shape of his body; it depended instead on the sensual pleasure he was feeling. The interviewer commented that she had never seen a man—including professional models and designers—who dressed more exquisitely.

"I have seen so much pain," this survivor replied, "in my life, so much ugliness and suffering. Here is one way I can bring a little beauty into the life of everyone I pass. It is the least I can do."

I still remember the exact corner I was passing on Westwood Boulevard when this interview aired on my car radio. I thought, How I wish I'd heard this man when I was fourteen. His was the kind of example that could change a person's life.

12

GAINING POWER

Becoming Agents for Change

The most powerful tool most of us possess is
our own voice.
    —Joyce Maynard, *At Home in the World*

THE LIGHTS DIM. A spotlight comes on, and a full-figured
woman in body-hugging black struts onto the stage. She is in
her mid-thirties, with a wide, open face surrounded by festoons
of dark curls, and as she lifts the microphone her brown eyes
sweep the audience of young professionals. She waits for the
chatter of mostly female voices to subside, then grins and shouts
her trick question: "Who's feeling fat today?"

Embarrassed laughter ripples across the room. Hands inch up
here and there. Onstage, Jessica Weiner pushes for more.
"Who's asked your boyfriend or husband if you look fat? Who's
complained to a girlfriend that you feel fat?" Soon the audito-
rium is pulsing with arms.

"Well, I have news for you," the voice booms from the stage.
"Fat is *not* a feeling!" Jessica lets that sink in, then gentles her
tone. She is irrepressible and fed up, but she is also sensitive to
the realities of women's lives. "When we say we feel fat, what

we really mean is 'Listen, pay attention' or 'You've angered and disappointed me.' Those are hard things for women to say, but we have to stop hiding our truth under the language of fat."

I first saw Jessica in action at a 2005 meeting of the National Eating Disorders Association, where she was publicizing her memoir, *A Very Hungry Girl*, and emceeing in her capacity as the association's goodwill ambassador. Her presence was huge, even before she spoke. Everyone in the room could feel her. That presence was not a function of her physical size but of her confidence. She didn't shrink from the spotlight or from herself. Instead, her personality seemed to expand to fill the space that connected her to her audience. She used her body instead of denying it. And this was just one of several hundred appearances she would make that year—when she wasn't running her media company, Parallax Entertainment, developing message-driven television shows, or turning out her advice column for girls on the Mary-Kate and Ashley Olsen Web site. Watching this young crusader in action, I found it impossible to picture her ever subsisting on five hundred calories a day. *The Hollywood Reporter* had anointed her "the next Oprah Winfrey," and she more than lives up to the comparison. With her big hair, her big eyes, and a laugh that fills the room, she has clearly made living large as life her personal specialty.

In fact, that disconnect between image and reality is central to her message. As she admits in her memoir, even during the seven years when she was routinely fasting and abusing laxatives, "I never looked sick or remotely like Kate Moss or Tracey Gold. . . . It seemed that no matter how hard I tried, my body fought back and refused to budge from a size and shape that I would one day recognize as healthy and functioning." For Jessica to get down to the size 9 that she wore throughout high school required the same compulsive insults to her body that might force another seventeen-year-old to a size 4. Her physical shape and size are as much a function of genetics as are the drive and organizational talents that helped Jessica launch her first company, a summer youth arts program, at twenty-one, and her first repertory company, ACT OUT, a year later. Since gaining control of her own eating disorder fifteen years ago, she's stopped fighting her body and started to use it, turning the self-loathing that infused her youth into fodder for her career as a self-described "actionist." She has made it her mission to expose America's hidden hungers and remove the taboo against satisfying them.

Jessica's transformation began in college. Eating disorders at any size, she realized in the support group she attended while an undergraduate at Penn State, are a signal of something that is wrong not just with one individual but with society. "If I didn't do something, I'd have to live with the consequences of a world that told women to stay inside and be quiet sexual objects."

She created a performance piece using the story of her own eating disorder and showcased it for her fellow students. Afterward, so many of her classmates came up to her—even girls who looked perfectly together—and confessed that they had the same problems, the same feelings and fears, that Jessica felt she'd found her calling. "As an artist," she wrote, "I was in heaven knowing that my creations had spanned an experience that many felt had moved them enough to speak out loud. As a human being, I was honored that others respected, and resonated with, my thoughts and experiences. For a girl who had been so hungry for attention, acceptance, understanding, love, peace, and connection, I was finally filled up in a way that I'd never imagined."

After college, as she toured with her ensemble, Jessica broadened her message to encompass issues of self-esteem, substance abuse, date rape, homophobia, peer pressure, child abuse, and leadership. Most of her audiences received her as warmly as that first one back at Penn State. Occasionally, however, she met active, hostile resistance. She made one particularly memorable solo appearance before a large audience of student athletes in a Midwestern college town where a star basketball player had just been arrested for stalking and raping a fellow student. Jessica had been brought in by two of the school's coaches to lead a mandatory student assembly about the implications of the arrest. She found herself facing four hundred student athletes who wanted no part of her message—or her. The male students loudly commented on her breasts, called her a bitch, complained that the school was forcing them to be there. The female students giggled as if these insults were brilliant and joked about the rape that had precipitated this session. For forty-five minutes Jessica tried to get through to them. Finally she began telling her own story of being sexually assaulted. One of her hecklers interrupted, "Someone needs to slap that bitch again and get her to shut up." When the two coaches, the only other adults present, did nothing, Jessica managed as much dignity as she could salvage. "If the way you treated me here tonight as a guest is the way you treat people in your community, then you're creating one sick place to live. You have wasted my time tonight, and I have nothing more to say to you." And with that, she walked out on the assembly.

How, I wondered, did she come back after an assault like that? How did she sustain faith in herself and her message? This was exactly the kind of brutality that had caused so many of us to take refuge in our eating disorders, to withdraw to our psychological corners and punish ourselves for what others had done to us. Jessica instead had kept going—indeed, had intensified her crusade to change the way young Americans treat each other.

"Those people aren't my higher power," she told me. "Those people don't define who I am. Was I devastated? Did I hurt? Did I question my purpose? Hell, yes. But I did what I always do to get by. First, I let myself feel it. I cried a lot. I was in a funk for a couple of days. But then I go to therapy. I pray. I meditate. I talk to people. I am loving to myself. I don't throw myself under the bus just because somebody else wants me to." She reflected for a few seconds. "When I receive such a direct spewing of hate and disrespect, I also look for the spiritual lesson in it. I try to break it down and not just say, I'm a total failure. What could I have done differently? That particular night, there were no teachers present. I was poorly set up and there were too many students. I also should have shifted my message to reach that particular audience. But I kept reminding myself, I have worked too damn hard and fought too damn hard to allow this kind of ignorance and hate to derail me."

One of the lessons Jessica's work has taught her is that those who most vehemently reject her messages of self-esteem and mutual respect are often those who feel too trapped or frightened to change. She was thinking of the girls in that college audience laughing along with the boys, and of one particular young woman who had walked out of one of her early performances only to appear several years later at another, standing and admitting that she had been actively bulimic and also abusing laxatives and diet pills when she first saw Jess. "I really hated you for showing me my life," the young woman told her. "But in the end you saved it."

To Jessica's thinking, however, that student had saved her own life. Jess simply showed her the truth. "Your recovery is none of my business, even if you're my mother or my best friend or my sister. I can care for you and support and hold a vision for you to be better and feel better, but your individual connection to your recovery and your life is your business." This principle of personal accountability is central to both Jessica's message and her survival as an activist. Her job as she sees it is to offer motivation, but she is not responsible for other people's choices and actions. She is not responsible for their heckling or ignoring her, nor is she responsible for "saving" them. What she is accountable for—always—are her own choices and actions, for keeping herself healthy, for moving forward, and for making sure that her work and words reflect her truest beliefs.

The paradox is that everyone and every action somehow connect, so each change Jessica makes in her own life inevitably has an impact on the people around her. The way she sees it, if every person she touches reaches out to others, soon millions of women could inspire one another to break free of their body obsessions. Just imagine what all that liberated talent and drive could accomplish! The possibilities, I agreed, were dazzling. If we'd all stop judging ourselves by the artificial standards of size and weight, we might be more effective in fighting other destructive judgments, such as racial and class discrimination. If we quit obsessing about the size of our thighs, we might be able to focus on the size of the national—or at least our household—debt. If we learned to express our power instead of suppressing it, we would reduce our own vulnerability to sexual abuse and set a vital example for our children. If we learned to defend our rights instead of minimizing them, we could demand the political respect that women, as half of humanity, deserve but too often are denied. When we become truly accountable for ourselves, we can't help but become more compassionate toward others. This was the essence of Jessica's one-woman campaign.

The challenge, she told me, is to avoid getting locked into any single objective or bogged down by any single obstacle. "Change is a process, like at a dinner party where you first let other people talk and all you do is listen, and then you form an opinion, and eventually you jump on board the conversation, and the next thing you know the discussion has progressed and you have to stop and listen again before moving on. I don't look at there ever being one end result. God willing, I am going to do lots of different things throughout my life and have lots of conversations. That's the great adventure."

Jessica left me with one important point, which not only underscored why she had chosen her particular career but echoed a sentiment I've heard from almost every person I've ever met who has recovered from anorexia or bulimia. "I have faith that I didn't die on the path I was on with my eating disorder," she said, "because I was supposed to use my life differently."

Gratitude, compassion, and a sense of purpose, I've come to believe, are as essential for health as calories. These traits can transform a history of private loss into gains that acquire transcendent weight and meaning, and this transcendence completes us in a way that even fully and confidently inhabiting our bodies alone cannot. The women and men I have met while writing this book are not out to single-handedly transform the world. Indeed, few are as public or outspoken as Jessica in their activism. But they are unanimous in their desire to make use of their experience, in small ways and large, and to serve as agents for change.

Personality, more than anything else, seems to shape the ways each individual channels this desire. Outgoing and dramatic, Jessica chose the stage as her platform. Writing, editing, and the arts appealed to those of us who were more introverted but wanted to inspire others to find their voice. Those with a more scientific or analytic bent became therapists, doctors, or researchers in the search for new treatments for psychological and medical disorders. Still others chose to work within their communities as teachers, librarians, or ministers. People with histories of eating disorders tend to be a driven lot, but the more self-aware we become, the less self-involved our preoccupations tend to be. Instead of working overtime to stifle our emotions and suppress our appetites, most of us these days are striving to make our lives significant.

While significance can still seem to me a dauntingly tall order, I try to remind myself that meaning and beauty reside even in random gestures. The secret to significance is simply to pay closer attention to whatever is happening right now. I am thinking as I write this of a conversation I had recently that would have been unimaginable to me when I was still in anorexic retreat. Indeed, it would have been unlikely even when I was forty. But lately I've been working to drop the defenses—those glasslike barriers—with which I've shielded myself most of my life; and so last winter I found myself in a small Vermont town chatting about midlife medical ailments with the postmistress, a woman in her sixties with a tight brown permanent and American flag pin on her breast. She was weighing and stamping my package when suddenly she began to cry. And for once I didn't turn away. I didn't worry about saying the wrong thing. I didn't fear getting involved with a stranger or just stand there feeling helpless. Instead, as no one else was in the post office, I rounded the counter to comfort her. Soon she was telling me that she had lost four members of her family to various diseases over the past year. I responded by telling her about my family's recent loss of my thirty-six-year-old niece to cancer. We talked for about fifteen minutes, letting out our mutual grief and consoling each other now among the risered mail slots and bins of outgoing letters. Then we shared a long, hard hug. There was no larger purpose to those fifteen minutes than compassion. That was precisely what made them significant.

"When I feel powerful," Yvonne Anderson, the theology professor, told me, "it's still so easy for me to withdraw from that feeling. Power brings a sense of possibility, of ownership, of responsibility. Being afraid of one's own power is central to anorexia and bulimia—even that word power-*full*." What sustains Yvonne is the knowledge, gained through experience, that the most comforting and comfortable source of power within herself is her ability to support and inspire others. She extends this support through her study and teaching. "The phrase that I love at the end of the Eucharistic prayer is 'O gentle God of resurrection—power.' The gentleness goes along with power. True power is about being able to empower others."

No one alive is beyond hope, and everyone alive has the power to inspire meaningful change. This is Yvonne's spiritual belief. It is mine as a writer. It is Jessica Weiner's as a performer and "actionist," Carolyn Costin's as an eating disorders therapist, and Sally Malloy's in her efforts to spread and study the benefits of mindfulness. Few of the women I interviewed, however, had come as close to losing hope as Cindy Bitter, a fifty-two-year-old anorexia veteran who serendipitously e-mailed me just as I was completing my research. For twenty-five years Cindy's average weight had been 70 pounds. Ultimately, all of her doctors but her psychotherapist had given up on her. Her long odyssey back to health had convinced her, she wrote, that "women with eating disorders who are attempting recovery desperately need to hear (and believe!) that not only is this disorder possible to overcome but that they can absolutely regain their health and their lives. I am living proof!"

The photographs Cindy attached to her message showed a pixie of a woman with a broad smile and warm brown hair cut short with bangs. She was hiking in Sedona in one picture, in the other mugging for the camera at a dinner party with her husband, a bearded, friendly-looking man who she later told me is an engineer with Xerox. *Radiant* was the word that came to mind as I studied these images of normalcy; and when I called her, that same radiance carried over the phone. Thirteen years after recovering, she still sounded surprised and delighted to report, "I wasn't lost, I was just deep inside."

Cindy's childhood never prepared her for the life she is leading today. Her parents were blue-collar Italian-Americans, lapsed Protestants with high school educations. Cindy grew up assuming she would marry young and build her life around her children, as her mother had. But her life began to follow a different course after an older girl across the street sexually molested her at age eleven. Timid, threatened, and ashamed, Cindy told no one. Depression sideswiped her at twelve. A year later her father was diagnosed with bipolar disorder. The constellation of losses expanded as her older sister left home, and by fourteen Cindy was anorexic. By eighteen she carried just 59 pounds on her five-foot-one frame. "I was lucky," she told me. "In those days, insurance paid for long-term treatment and didn't restrict my doctors. I was in and out of hospitals, anywhere from three to thirteen months at a time, for fifteen years. That kept me alive until I was able to get better."

Cindy was thirty-three when she finally reached her turning point. "I missed me—the little girl I remembered before the depression. I had become so afraid of being afraid. I knew I should have been dead. And then my brother came for a visit. It sounds crazy because we were not a churchgoing family, but he said God had come to him in a dream and told him, 'She's going to be okay.' I believed him. And then I had this thought out of the blue: if I'm going to be okay, I want to go to college. Where did *that* come from! I didn't even know who I was, but I made this my goal. I chose to get better from that point on."

It took seven more years, during which Cindy, like Jessica, discovered that her long siege of loss had endowed her with a gift that she could offer to others through her story. First, her doctors asked her to return to the hospital to talk with medical students about her progress. Then eating disorder organizations began asking her to speak. The simple fact that she had survived, she realized, was a source of hope and inspiration to others. She wrote and self-published a memoir and continued occasionally speaking even as she began to turn her life in new directions. She earned her college degree in health sciences, and by age forty she was working as a career coach for people recovering from brain injuries.

The kinship she felt with her clients went beyond empathy. When she learned that the brain recovers from injury by creating new neural pathways to compensate for the damaged areas, it struck her that the same process was occurring during her own recuperation. This was why it had taken so long for her to feel normal. "My disorder was a path I'd created early on and worn through use into a superhighway. It seemed like the only way I had to go. But it only led one place, and that was death. Recovery was all about clearing new paths to healthier destinations, using them and reusing them until these new roads were as wide open as the old, disordered one. If I stayed off that old highway long enough, it would get so overgrown it wasn't accessible anymore. That's why recovery was so hard at first, but also why it got easier and easier as I kept at it."

The one loss that Cindy had reconciled herself to never regaining was her face. During the long decades of her eating disorder, her body had cannibalized her bones to the extent that her skull had lost its natural contours. Her cheekbones had flattened. Her jaws had thinned. She'd lost all her teeth. Even after her weight was back up to 110 pounds (matching her mother and sister, who were also five foot one), her facial bones continued weakening until she could not even wear dentures. Surgeon after surgeon told her there was nothing to be done. She was stunned when, at forty-nine, she met a maxillofacial specialist who was willing to try to rebuild her face to match the structure she'd last had at seventeen. The series of procedures took eighteen months. There were complications. She had to take a leave from work. But as her original image of herself physically reemerged, she felt she had to find a new way to express her gratitude and extend it to others. Those she could help the most, she realized, were those struggling with the same terrors that had nearly cost her her life.

"When I talked to audiences of eating disorder patients, the same questions kept coming. How do I recover right? What happens after treatment?" Cindy found that women would get lost or stuck in between old and new habits, sometimes years after regaining their normal weight. The same perfectionism that had made them sick would strangle their attempts to get better as they worried that there was a right way or wrong way to improve, that they would need some sort of scale to measure their return to health, the same way they used to measure their weight, that there was some ideal state they had to attain in order to qualify as "recovered." Cindy began "life coaching" small groups of these women in transition and found that she understood how to help them expand and navigate their own new roads to health while steering them clear of their old self-destructive habits. "I liken it to helping them learn to drive forward. A therapist spends a lot of time helping people accurately read the rearview mirror, but I concentrate on what's in front of the windshield. What do you see? Where do you want to go? How fast should you travel, and how do you talk and feel and think and drive at the same time? How do you correct if you make a wrong turn, then learn from your mistakes? I get them to think about what's possible and to believe in themselves, that they can go anywhere they set their minds to. They just have to make the decision to move forward. And then I stay with them until they're familiar with the new roads and until the safer driving habits become automatic."

I asked Cindy, now that she had regained her health, if she had found a way to make peace with the years she'd lost to anorexia. "Of course!" she exclaimed. "They're part of who I am. I'm so *proud* of being recovered. I'm happy all the time now, but I know I couldn't be this happy if I hadn't been so sad."

"Out of despair, joy," John Milton wrote in *Paradise Lost*. The lesson is as old as Genesis. We cannot gain wisdom without losing our innocence. Without hunger there can be no satisfaction. Recovery, then, is like alchemy. It turns grief for a missing sister or brother into a source of strength. Shame over an early childhood trauma yields compassion and confidence. Fear shape-shifts into hope. The transformation does not make us flawless but richer for our flaws. And as Cindy said, regret plays no role in this.

Denial of pain, remember, is the reason we develop eating disorders. True health, by contrast, means accepting that no human being or experience can ever be uniformly or "perfectly" happy. No one, as Jessica put it, has "a hall pass to skip all the shitty stuff." That shitty stuff, from the teasing we endured in grade school, to midlife losses of friends and lovers, to our physical decline into old age, is an essential part of what makes us who we are. To ignore, suppress, or spend our lives regretting our hardships is to diminish ourselves.

I believe that the greatest asset any of us possesses is our own life story. The sum of all we've experienced and learned, of everyone we've ever known, everything we've ever accomplished, and everywhere we've ever been, our story is the one belonging that grows with each passing day and that we can share without limit. But to realize the full power and dimension of this treasure, we have to be willing to tell the whole truth. This is a lesson that I've learned with considerable reluctance, as a daughter, wife, mother, and friend, and also professionally as a writer. While I would never say that I've mastered this lesson, in my fifteen years as a novelist, my work has forced me to recognize that any story without conflict between good and evil, highs and lows, and both losses and gains is not only boring but false. Characters whose sole traits are their beautiful skin and size-2 Armani wardrobes might as well be paper dolls. Real human beings are richer and more complex than the greatest literary character ever created. Anna Karenina and Jane Eyre have nothing on Hannah Winters, with her string of suicide attempts and passionate motherhood, or Irene Slocum, vanquishing anorexia while single-handedly raising four children out of rural poverty, or Cindy Bitters reclaiming her face at forty-nine.

Whether our forte is galloping racehorses, designing houses, or running a theater company, we all have surprising talents. Whether we binge, purge, shoplift, smoke, drink, brood, or bite our fingernails, we all have vices. And whether we resemble Kathy Bates or Jennifer Lopez, Oprah Winfrey or Jessica Simpson, we all can find fault with some aspect of our looks and our lives. It's what we do with our faults, as well as with our talents and circumstances, that reveals our character. A teenager chooses to starve herself not simply because she has been molested, because her mother doesn't understand her, or because she is hypersensitive or wishes she could look like Cameron Diaz. She punishes herself for any or all these reasons, but also for at least one more: she punishes herself for being human. Healing occurs when she dares to replace punishment with acceptance and understanding.

But how will I know it's happening? This is the question Cindy Bitter hears most often. She recalled her very first client, a young woman named Melissa, saying, "I want to gain back my life, but when does recovery start?"

Cindy took Melissa's hand. "It's already started," she told her. "It's happening. This is your life. Now."

As I come to the end of this book, I have to admit that I'm still gaining, in all the best senses of the word. Thanks to love, friendship, taste, touch, children, marriage, therapy, walking, meditation, leisurely swims, writing, reading, and an abundance of other joys, my eating disorders are behind me. I sincerely doubt I will ever succumb to their lure again. Curious as it may sound, one reason is that I now respect the traits that make me vulnerable to these disorders. Developing the skills, strategies, and regimens to manage these traits is a lifelong process. Yet I would not want to be "cured" of these qualities, any more than I would want to be cured of my heritage or my memories. The fact is, everyone's past contains both wonderful and awful memories. Everyone's family contains some delightful and some impossible relatives. That mix and contrast are as essential to human identity as lightness and darkness are to a photograph. Becoming self-aware and self-confident enough to avoid psychological traps such as eating disorders means more than controlling the contradictions within our own nature. It means, in a deep and honest way, appreciating them.

In reaching this conclusion, I've changed the way I think about recovery. I no longer define it in relation to illness but as an ongoing process of *restoration and discovery*. I see now that I am continuously restoring the essential individual I was born to be while discovering my unfolding connection to the world around me. This process, especially at this late stage of my life, has far more to do with growing than healing, though both will always be involved. And there will be setbacks. Sometimes it will seem as if I'm making no progress but simply repeating myself, turning around and around the same old habits and ways of thinking. But as long as I can feel myself present, open and awake, I know I am gradually gaining.

In her memoir, Karen Armstrong likened this process to climbing a narrow spiral staircase: "I tried to get off it and join others on what seemed to me to be a broad, noble flight of steps, thronged with people. But I kept falling off, and when I went back to my own twisting stairwell I found a fulfillment that I had not expected. Now I have to mount my staircase alone." This, for better and for worse, is the ultimate truth about recovery: Each of us must find our own path. We must dare to follow it even when others can't understand or don't approve. And we must each take our own sweet time to savor all that we gain as we move outward, into and through the richness of life that awaits us.

Acknowledgments

Writing this book has been an education—and I mean that literally. In the early stages of research for *Gaining*, I realized that my eating disorder had left a number of holes in my life that, thirty years later, remained unfilled. One of the biggest gaps was educational. In college, I had been too afraid of failure to risk Yale's serious literature courses. I had been too introverted to risk a writing course that would have pushed me to expose myself honestly. And even when emerging from anorexia in my twenties, I still lacked sufficient faith in my abilities to consider seeking a graduate degree. I let my fears dictate my choices instead of choosing to overrule those fears. Now I decided to change that lifelong pattern. Even at fifty, I realized, it wasn't too late to take on Dante and T. S. Eliot, Virginia Woolf and Henry James. Nor was it too late to stretch my own writing in new directions. The depth of knowledge I stood to gain would grant me the confidence to teach others. So I applied to the Bennington College MFA Program in Writing and Literature. In 2004 I began working toward a master's in nonfiction, with *Gaining* as my thesis. Over the next two years I had the privilege and the pleasure of studying with Sven Birkerts, Susan Cheever, Tom Bissell, Ben Cheever, and Bob Shacochis. Their intellectual rigor, curiosity, good humor, and encouragement have enriched this book in more ways than I can count. More important, they have pushed me to ask the tough questions of myself; to think deeply about who I am, what I want and believe, and why; and to always write the truth to the best of my ability. I owe heartfelt thanks as well to my classmates for their caring honesty and to Bennington Writing Seminars director Liam Rector and associate director Priscilla Hodgkins for their gracious orchestration of the music within "the vortex."

The women and men who generously shared their stories for this book were teachers of a different kind. Although my promise to protect their privacy prevents me from naming them, I want to acknowledge all that they have taught me about resilience and courage and hard-won wisdom. It wasn't always easy for them to connect the dots of pain and fear and resilience within their own lives, but their collective insights prove that knowledge really is power. It is impossible to resolve a distress signal like anorexia or bulimia without looking squarely at the true source of distress. The ability of these individuals to unflinchingly confront and overcome the obstacles that once held them back will, I hope and trust, empower others to do the same.

I owe a similar vote of thanks to the many researchers and therapists whose work and words dramatically changed my understanding of eating disorders—and myself—over the three years I spent writing this book. I am particularly grateful for the time, support, and advice given me by Drs. Kelly Brownell, Mary Kay Cocharo, Carolyn Costin, David Herzog, Walter Kaye, Lisa Lilenfeld, Deborah Lynn, Margo Maine, Sheila Reindl, Susan Smalley, Michael Strober, Janet Treasure, Mark Warren, Tiffany Rush-Wilson, and Joel Yager.

I would also like to express my gratitude to Lisa See, for introducing me to China's "lovesick maidens"; Jack Miles, for prompting me to explore the spiritual aspects of eating disorders and for taking the time to help me see how society and religion often "employ affliction"; Deborah Jones, for reading the earliest chapters and offering invaluable encouragement and inspiration; and Carolyn Hall-Young and Warren Young, for embodying love and wonder. Michael Gold tragically died as I was finishing this book. He taught me to recognize and savor the best that life has to offer, and I will always remember him as a dazzling star.

The evolution of every book has its ups and downs, and this book proved no exception. For their faith in me, yet again, I must thank my agent, Richard Pine, as well as Lori Andiman; my publisher, Jamie Raab; and my patient and gifted editor, Caryn Karmatz Rudy.

Finally, I want to thank my family. My parents have not always understood my choices and decisions in life, but their love for me has been a constant that I cling to and return, amplified by gratitude and admiration. Graham and Dan have been so tolerant over the years, as I've disappeared into my office and thoughts, prodded them and their friends for perspectives to test my own, and generally burdened them with the dubious distinction of having a mother who writes. I adore and admire them both.

As for Marty, I have three words: *love—honor—joy*. I owe you everything I hold dear.

Appendix I

RESOURCES FOR INFORMATION AND ACTIVISM

For general information about eating disorders and treatment:

The Academy for Eating Disorders (www.aedweb.org) is an international professional organization that promotes research, treatment, and prevention of eating disorders. The AED provides education, training, and a forum for collaboration and professional dialogue.

Anorexia Nervosa and Related Eating Disorders (www.anred .com) is a nonprofit organization that provides information about anorexia nervosa, bulimia nervosa, binge eating disorder, and other less-well-known food and weight disorders.

The Eating Disorder Referral and Information Center (www.edreferral.com) offers referrals to eating disorder specialists, treatment facilities, and support groups, and provides educational resources.

Gürze Books (www.gurze.com) publishes and distributes a wide variety of books, videos, and periodicals about eating disorders and related therapies.

The National Association of Anorexia Nervosa and Associated Disorders (www.anad.org) is the oldest national nonprofit organization dedicated to alleviating the problems of eating disorders and promoting healthy lifestyles.

The National Eating Disorders Association (www.na tionaleatingdisorders.org) works to expand public understanding and prevention of eating disorders; advocates for access to quality treatment; and offers support for families through education, advocacy, and research.

The National Eating Disorder Information Centre (www .nedic.ca) is a Canadian nonprofit organization that provides information and resources on eating disorders and weight preoccupation.

Something Fishy (www.something-fishy.org) is a pro-recovery website founded by Amy Medina, who herself has a history of anorexia, and her husband, Tony. The site hosts chat forums and links to a wide array of information sources.

For information about specific therapies described in this book:

Dialectic Behavior Therapy (DBT) and
Cognitive Behavior Therapy (CBT)

The Association for Behavioral and Cognitive Therapies (www.aabt.org), a professional organization, produces books, videos, and tapes about available therapies and offers a referral service of qualified therapists.

The Behavioral Research and Therapy Clinics (www.brtc .psych.washington.edu) is a clinical research and training center, located at the University of Washington, Seattle, where psychotherapeutic treatments for severe and chronic personality disorders are developed and evaluated. Dialectical Behavior Therapy was developed here by the BRTC's director, Dr. Marsha M. Linehan.

The Maudsley Method
(also called family-based treatment)

The Eating Disorders Program at the University of Chicago Hospitals (www.psychiatry.uchicago.edu/clinical/clinics/edp) offers comprehensive treatment for eating disorders. The program is directed by Dr. Daniel le Grange, who helped develop family-based treatment for anorexia nervosa while completing his clinical training at London's Maudsley Hospital. He is the coauthor, with James Lock, of *Help Your Teenager Beat an Eating Disorder*, an excellent overview of this new treatment approach.

Equine Assisted Psychotherapy

The Equine Assisted Growth and Learning Association (www .eagala.org) is a nonprofit organization that offers information about the emerging field of Equine Assisted Psychotherapy.

Mindfulness
(also called mindful awareness)

UCLA's Mindful Awareness Research Center (www.marc .ucla.edu) was created to study the psychological, medical, educational, and social benefits of mindful awareness—"the moment-by-moment process of actively observing, and drawing inferences from one's physical, mental, and emotional experiences"—for children, adolescents, and adults. The center also evaluates various mindfulness practices, such as meditation, yoga, tai chi, and chi gong, in clinical and nonclinical settings and offers information and resources for the general public.

The University of Massachusetts's Center for Mindfulness in Medicine, Health Care, and Society (www.umassmed.edu/cfm) conducts clinical research and offers education and practical training in mindfulness. Its initiatives include the country's oldest and largest academic medical center-based program for stress reduction.

For information about public health and insurance policies that relate to eating disorders:

The Eating Disorders Coalition for Research, Policy, & Action (www.eatingdisorderscoalition.org) works to raise awareness of eating disorders as a public health priority and to increase resources for improved research, education, prevention, and treatment of these disorders.

For help in teaching children to have a healthy body image:

About-Face (www.About-Face.org) is a San Francisco-based group that challenges the media's idealization of female thinness and employs education and activism to promote positive self-esteem in girls and women of all sizes, races, and backgrounds.

Dads & Daughters (www.DadsAndDaughters.org) is a national educational and advocacy organization that provides tools to strengthen father-daughter relationships and works to change cultural messages to encourage girls to care less about how they look and more about what they do, think, or feel.

How you can help expand our understanding of eating disorders:

The National Institute of Health and the National Institute of Mental Health (www.angenetics.org) are currently funding groundbreaking research into the genetics of anorexia nervosa. The study is seeking families in which two or more relatives (sisters, brothers, cousins, aunts, grandparents) currently have anorexia or have had it in the past. If your family fits this description, please consider participating in this important research. The study's ten sites are located throughout North America and Europe. For more information, call 1-888-895-3886 (toll free) or e-mail: edresearch@msx.upmc.edu.

Appendix II

SUGGESTIONS FOR PARENTS

With thanks to Kelly Brownell, Ph.D.,
professor and chair of psychology and director,
Yale Center for Eating and Weight Disorders

If you are concerned that your child may be developing or has an eating disorder, be proactive!

- Learn as much as you can about eating disorders. An excellent book is *Helping Your Child Overcome an Eating Disorder: What You Can Do at Home* by Bethany A. Teachman and colleagues (Oakland, CA: New Harbinger Publications, 2003).
- Work with school officials. Contact the school counseling office or the office of the dean of students (or the equivalent). Do not fear that this will tarnish your child's record. College and secondary school administrators understand that adolescence is a time of stress and sometimes distress. Their job is to help students stay safe and healthy and make the most of their educations.
- Make sure your child receives optimal help. College counseling services vary. While these services are staffed by professionals who understand the general health care needs of college students, they are not always knowledgeable on the

up-to-date treatments for eating disorders. Typically students are allowed a limited number of counseling sessions. If the care does not seem adequate, call the psychology department of your child's college or consult Appendix I for referrals to local eating disorder specialists.

- If the problem is severe and your child is away at school, consider having her take a leave of absence and return home during treatment. The stress of school can make it difficult for a student to focus on recovery. Consult your child's principal, dean, or headmaster and discuss the available options with your child in order to decide the best course of action.

- Remember that recovery requires patience and compassion. An eating disorder may subside, flare up again, or take a different form. Throughout this difficult process, the love, support, and understanding of the whole family will be tremendously important to your child.

Selected Bibliography

Allaz, Anne-Françoise, Martine Bernstein, Patrick Rouget, Marc Archinard, and Alfredo Morabia. "Body Weight Preoccupation in Middle-Age and Ageing Women: A General Population Survey." *International Journal of Eating Disorders* 23 (April 1998): 287–94.

Anderluh, Maria Brecelj, Kate Tchanturia, Sophia Rabe-Hesketh, and Janet Treasure. "Childhood Obsessive-Compulsive Personality Traits in Adult Women with Eating Disorders: Defining a Broader Eating Disorder Phenotype." *American Journal of Psychiatry* 160 (February 2003): 242–47.

Andersen, Arnold E. "Progress in Eating Disorders Research." *American Journal of Psychiatry* 158 (April 2001): 515–17.

Armstrong, Karen. *The Spiral Staircase: My Climb Out of Darkness*. New York: Anchor Books, 2005. First published in 2004 by Alfred A. Knopf.

Becker, Anne E., Debra L. Franko, Alexandra Speck, and David B. Herzog. "Ethnicity and Differential Access to Care for Eating Disorder Symptoms." *International Journal of Eating Disorders* 33 (March 2003): 205–12.

Bell, Rudolph M. *Holy Anorexia*. Chicago: University of Chicago Press, 1985.

Beresin, Eugene, Christopher Gordon, and David Herzog. "The

Process of Recovering from Anorexia Nervosa." In *Psycho-analysis and Eating Disorders*, edited by Jules R. Bemporad and David B. Herzog. New York: Guilford Press, 1989.

Bordo, Susan. *Unbearable Weight: Feminism, Western Culture, and the Body*, 10th ed. Berkeley: University of California Press, 2004.

Brewerton, Timothy. "The Role of Traumatic Experiences." *Eating Disorders Today*. Winter 2006: 1ff.

Brownell, Kelly D., and Katherine Battle Horgen. *Food Fight: The Inside Story of the Food Industry, America's Obesity Crisis, and What We Can Do About It*. Chicago: Contemporary Books, 2004.

Bruch, Hilde. *The Golden Cage: The Enigma of Anorexia Nervosa*. Cambridge: Harvard University Press, 2001. First published in 1978 by Harvard University Press.

Brumberg, Joan Jacobs. *Fasting Girls: The Emergence of Anorexia Nervosa as a Modern Disease*. Cambridge: Harvard University Press, 1988.

————. *Fasting Girls: The History of Anorexia Nervosa*. New York: Vintage, 2000.

Bulik, Cynthia M., and Kenneth S. Kendler. "'I Am What I (Don't) Eat': Establishing an Identity Independent of an Eating Disorder." *American Journal of Psychiatry* 157 (November 2000): 1755–60.

————, Patrick F. Sullivan, Jennifer L. Fear, and Alison Pickering. "Outcome of Anorexia Nervosa: Eating Attitudes, Personality, and Parental Bonding." *International Journal of Eating Disorders* 28 (September 2000): 139–47.

————, Patrick F. Sullivan, Jennifer L. Fear, Alison Pickering, Aria Dawn, and Mandy McCullin. "Fertility and Reproduction in Women with Anorexia Nervosa: A Controlled Study." *Journal of Clinical Psychiatry* 60 (February 1999): 130–35.

————, Frederica Tozzi, Charles Anderson, Suzanne E. Mazzeo, Steve Aggen, and Patrick F. Sullivan. "The Relation Between Eating Disorders and Components of Perfectionism." *American Journal of Psychiatry* 160 (February 2003): 366–68.

Chernin, Kim. *The Hungry Self: Women, Eating and Identity*. New York: HarperPerennial, 1994. First published in 1985 by Times Books.

————. *The Obsession: Reflections on the Tyranny of Slenderness*. New York: HarperPerennial, 1994. First published in 1981 by Harper & Row.

Cloninger, Robert. *Feeling Good: The Science of Well-Being*. New York: Oxford University Press, 2004.

Csikszentmihalyi, Mihaly. *Flow: The Psychology of Optimal Experience*. New York: Harper & Row, 1990.

Dansky, Bonnie S., Timothy D. Brewerton, Dean G. Kilpatrick, and Patrick M. O'Neil. "The National Women's Study: Relationship of Victimization and Posttraumatic Stress Disorder to Bulimia Nervosa." *International Journal of Eating Disorders* 21 (April 1997): 213–28.

Erikson, Erik H. *Identity, Youth, and Crisis*. New York: W. W. Norton, 1968.

Fairbairn, W. R. D. *Psychoanalytic Studies of the Personality*. New York: Routledge, 1994. First published in 1943 by Tavistock.

Fairburn, Christopher G., and Kelly D. Brownell, eds. *Eating Disorders and Obesity*, 2nd ed. New York: Guilford Press, 2002.

Faravelli, Carlo, Alice Giugni, Stefano Salvatori, and Valdo Ricca. "Psychopathology After Rape." *American Journal of Psychiatry* 161 (August 2004): 1483–85.

Finkelhor, David. "Current Information on the Scope and Nature of Child Sexual Abuse." *The Future of Children* 4, no. 2 (1994): 31–53.

Fisher, M. F. K. *The Gastronomical Me*. New York: North Point Press, 1989. First published in 1943 by Duell, Sloan, & Pearce.

Fonda, Jane. *My Life So Far*. New York: Random House, 2005.

Franko, Debra L., Mark A. Blais, Anne E. Becker, Sherrie Selwyn Delinsky, Dara N. Greenwood, Andrea T. Flores, Elizabeth R. Ekeblad, Kamryn T. Eddy, and David B. Herzog. "Pregnancy Complications and Neonatal Outcomes in Women with Eating Disorders." *American Journal of Psychiatry* 158 (September 2001): 1461–66.

Fromm, Erich. *To Have or to Be?* London and New York: Continuum, 2005. First published in 1976 by Harper & Row.

Gordon, Mary. *Pearl.* New York: Pantheon, 2005.

Gottlieb, Lori. *Stick Figure: A Diary of My Former Self.* New York: Berkley Books, 2001. First published in 2000 by Simon & Schuster.

Gray, Francine du Plessix. *Simone Weil.* New York: Viking, 2001.

Grice, D. E., K. A. Halmi, M. M. Fichter, M. Strober, D. B. Woodside, J. T. Treasure, A. S. Kaplan, P. J. Magistretti, D. Goldman, C. M. Bulik, W. H. Kaye, and W. H. Berrettini. "Evidence for a Susceptibility Gene for Anorexia Nervosa on Chromosome 1." *American Journal of Human Genetics* 70 (March 2002): 787.

Halmi, Katherine A., Suzanne R. Sunday, Kelly L. Klump, Michael Strober, James F. Leckman, Manfred Fichter, Allan Kaplan, Blake Woodside, Janet Treasure, Wade H. Berrettini, Mayadah Al Shabbout, Cynthia M. Bulik, and Walter H. Kaye. "Obsessions and Compulsions in Anorexia Nervosa Subtypes." *International Journal of Eating Disorders* 33 (April 2003): 308–19.

Hamsun, Knut. *Hunger.* Translated by Robert Bly. New York: Farrar, Straus, and Giroux, 1998. First published in 1890.

Harrison, Kathryn. *The Kiss.* New York: Random House, 1997.

––––––. *The Mother Knot.* New York: Random House, 2004.

Hornbacher, Marya. *Wasted: A Memoir of Anorexia and Bulimia.* New York: HarperCollins, 1998.

Johnson, Jeffrey, Patricia Cohen, Stephanie Kasen, and Judith S. Brook. "Childhood Adversities Associated with Risk for Eating Disorders or Weight Problems During Adolescence or Early Adulthood." *American Journal of Psychiatry* 159 (March 2002): 394–400.

Kaye, Walter H., Cynthia M. Bulik, Laura Thornton, Nicole Barbarich, Kim Masters, and the Price Foundation Collaborative Group. "Comorbidity of Anxiety Disorders with Anorexia and Bulimia Nervosa." *American Journal of Psychiatry* 161 (December 2004): 2215–21.

––––––, Catherine G. Greeno, Howard Moss, John Fernstrom,

Madelyn Fernstrom, Lila R. Lilenfeld, Theodore E. Weltzin, and J. John Mann. "Alterations in Serotonin Activity and Psychiatric Symptoms After Recovery from Bulimia Nervosa." *Archives of General Psychiatry* 55 (October 1998): 927–35.

Keel, Pamela, and James E. Mitchell. "Outcome in Bulimia Nervosa." *American Journal of Psychiatry* 154 (March 1997): 313–21.

Kendler, Kenneth S., and Xiao-Qing Liu, Charles O. Gardner, Michael E. McCullough, David Larson, and Carol A. Prescott. "Dimensions of Religiosity and Their Relationship to Lifetime Psychiatric and Substance Use Disorders." *American Journal of Psychiatry* 160 (March 2003): 496–503.

Klump, Kelly L., Cynthia M. Bulik, Christine Pollice, Katherine A. Halmi, Manfred M. Fichter, Wade H. Berrettini, Bernie Devlin, Michael Strober, Allan Kaplan, Blake Woodside, Janet Treasure, Mayadah Shabbout, Lisa R. R. Lilenfeld, Katherine H. Plotnicov, and Walter H. Kaye. "Temperament and Character in Women with Anorexia Nervosa." *Journal of Nervous and Mental Disease* 188 (September 2000).

———, Michael Strober, Cynthia M. Bulik, Laura Thornton, Craig Johnson, Bernie Devlin, Manfred M. Fichter, Katherine A. Halmi, Allan S. Kaplan, D. Blake Woodside, Scott Crow, James Mitchell, Alessandro Rotondo, Pamela K. Keel, Wade H. Berrettini, Katherine Plotnicov, Christine Pollice, Lisa R. Lilenfeld, and Walter H. Kaye. "Personality Characteristics of Women Before and After Recovery from an Eating Disorder." *Psychological Medicine* 34 (November 2004): 1407–18.

Knapp, Caroline. *Appetites: Why Women Want*. New York: Counterpoint, 2003.

———. *Drinking: A Love Story*. New York: Dial Press, 1996.

———. *The Merry Recluse: A Life in Essays*. New York: Counterpoint, 2004.

———. *Pack of Two: The Intricate Bond Between People and Dogs*. New York: Dial Press, 1998.

Kramer, Peter D. *Listening to Prozac*. New York: Penguin Books, 1997.

Leaska, Mitchell. *Granite and Rainbow: The Hidden Life of Virginia Woolf.* New York: Farrar, Straus, and Giroux, 1998.

Levenkron, Steven. *Anatomy of Anorexia.* New York: W. W. Norton, 2000.

Lilenfeld, Lisa R., Walter H. Kaye, Catherine G. Greeno, Kathleen R. Merikangas, Katherine Plotnicov, Christine Pollice, Radhika Rao, Michael Strober, Cynthia M. Bulik, and Linda Nagy. "A Controlled Study of Anorexia Nervosa and Bulimia Nervosa: Psychiatric Disorders in First-Degree Relatives and Effects of Proband Comorbidity." *Archives of General Psychiatry* 55 (July 1998): 603–10.

Linehan, Marsha M. *Cognitive-Behavioral Treatment of Borderline Personality Disorder.* New York: Guilford Press, 1993.

Lock, James. "Innovative Family-Based Treatment for Anorexia Nervosa." *The Brown University Child and Adolescent Behavior Letter* 17, no. 4 (April 2001).

———, and Daniel le Grange. *Help Your Teenager Beat an Eating Disorder.* New York: Guilford Press, 2005.

———, Daniel le Grange, W. Stewart Agras, and Christopher Dare. *Treatment Manual for Anorexia Nervosa: A Family-Based Approach.* New York: Guilford Press, 2001.

Matsunaga, Hisato, Walter H. Kaye, Claire McConaha, Katherine Plotnicov, Christine Pollice, and Radhiko Rao. "Personality Disorders Among Subjects Recovered from Eating Disorders." *International Journal of Eating Disorders* 27 (April 2000): 353–57.

Maychick, Diana. *Audrey Hepburn: An Intimate Portrait.* New York: Birch Lane Press, 1993.

Maynard, Joyce. *At Home in the World: A Memoir.* New York: Picador, 1998.

Morgan, C. D., M. W. Wiederman, and T. L. Pryor. "Sexual Functioning and Attitudes of Eating-Disordered Women: A Follow-up Study." *Journal of Sex & Marital Therapy* 21 (Summer 1995): 67–77.

Orbach, Susie. *Hunger Strike: The Anorectic's Struggle as a Metaphor for Our Age.* New York: W. W. Norton, 1986.

Orenstein, Peggy. *Schoolgirls: Young Women, Self-esteem, and the Confidence Gap*. New York: Anchor Books, 2000. First published in 1994 by Doubleday.

Paul, Thomas, Kirsten Schroeter, Bernhard Dahme, and Detlev O. Nutzinger. "Self-Injurious Behavior in Women with Eating Disorders." *American Journal of Psychiatry* 159 (March 2002): 408–11.

Pike, Kathleen M., B. Timothy Walsh, Kelly Vitousek, G. Terence Wilson, and Jay Bauer. "Cognitive Behavior Therapy in the Posthospitalization Treatment of Anorexia Nervosa." *American Journal of Psychiatry* 160 (November 2003): 2046–49.

Pipher, Mary. *Reviving Ophelia: Saving the Selves of Adolescent Girls*. New York: Putnam, 1994.

Rayworth, Beth B., Lauren A. Wise, and Bernard L. Harlow. "Childhood Abuse and Risk of Eating Disorders in Women." *Epidemiology* 15 (May 2004): 271–78.

Reiland, Rachel. *Get Me Out of Here: My Recovery from Borderline Personality Disorder*. Center City, MN: Hazelden, 2004.

Reindl, Sheila. *Sensing the Self: Women's Recovery from Bulimia*. Cambridge: Harvard University Press, 2001.

Safer, Debra L., Christy F. Tech, and W. Stewart Agras. "Dialectic Behavior Therapy for Bulimia Nervosa." *American Journal of Psychiatry* 158 (April 2001): 632–34.

Sartre, Jean-Paul. *Being and Nothingness*. New York: Washington Square Press, 1992. First published in 1943 by Gallimard.

Sollid, Charlotte, Kirsten Wisborg, Jakob Hjort, and Niels Jørgen Secher. "Eating Disorder That Was Diagnosed Before Pregnancy and Pregnancy Outcome." *American Journal of Obstetrics & Gynecology* 190 (January 2004): 206–10.

Solomon, Andrew. *The Noonday Demon: An Atlas of Depression*. New York: Scribner, 2001.

Srinivasagam, N. M., W. H. Kaye, K. H. Plotnicov, C. Greeno, T. E. Weltzin, and R. Rao. "Persistent Perfectionism, Symmetry, and Exactness After Long-term Recovery from Anorexia Nervosa." *American Journal of Psychiatry* 152 (November 1995): 1630–34.

Steiger, Howard, Lise Gauvin, Mimi Israël, N. M. K. Ng Ying Kin, Simon N. Young, and Julie Roussin. "Serotonin Function, Personality-Trait Variations, and Childhood Abuse in Women with Bulimia-Spectrum Eating Disorders." *Journal of Clinical Psychiatry* 65 (June 2004).

Stein, D., W. H. Kaye, H. Matsunaga, I. Orbach, D. Har-Even, G. Frank, C. W. McConaha, and R. Rao. "Eating-Related Concerns, Mood, and Personality Traits in Recovered Bulimia Nervosa Subjects: A Replication Study." *International Journal of Eating Disorders* 32 (September 2002): 225–29.

Steinhausen, Hans-Christoph. "The Outcome of Anorexia Nervosa in the 20th Century." *American Journal of Psychiatry* 159 (August 2002): 1284–93.

Strober, Michael, Roberta Freeman, Carlyn Lampert, Jane Diamond, and Walter Kaye. "Controlled Family Study of Anorexia Nervosa and Bulimia Nervosa: Evidence of Shared Liability and Transmission of Partial Syndromes." *American Journal of Psychiatry* 157 (March 2000): 393–401.

Sullivan, Patrick F., Cynthia M. Bulik, Jennifer L. Fear, and Alison Pickering. "Outcome of Anorexia Nervosa: A Case-Control Study." *American Journal of Psychiatry* 155 (July 1998): 939–46.

Vandereycken, Walter. "Families of Patients with Eating Disorders." In *Eating Disorders and Obesity: A Comprehensive Handbook,* edited by Christopher G. Fairburn and Kelly D. Brownell. New York: Guilford Press, 2002.

Viorst, Judith. *Imperfect Control: Our Lifelong Struggle with Power and Surrender.* New York: Free Press, 1999. First published by Simon & Schuster in 1998.

Wade, Tracey D., Cynthia M. Bulik, Michael Neale, and Kenneth S. Kendler. "Anorexia Nervosa and Major Depression: Shared Genetic and Environmental Risk Factors." *American Journal of Psychiatry* 157 (March 2000): 469–71.

Weiner, Jessica. *A Very Hungry Girl: How I Filled Up on Life—and How You Can Too!* Carlsbad, CA: Hay House, 2003.

Westen, Drew, and Jennifer Harnden-Fischer. "Personality Profiles in Eating Disorders: Rethinking the Distinction Between Axis I and Axis II." *American Journal of Psychiatry* 158 (April 2001): 547–62.

Winnicott, D. W. *Home Is Where We Start From: Essays by a Psycholanalyst.* New York: W. W. Norton, 1986.

Woodside, D. Blake, Cynthia M. Bulik, Laura Thornton, Kelly L. Klump, Federica Tozzi, Manfred M. Fichter, Katherine A. Halmi, Allan S. Kaplan, Michael Strober, Bernie Devlin, Silviu-Alin Bacanu, Kelly Ganjei, Scott Crow, James Mitchell, Alessandro Rotondo, Mauro Mauri, Giovanni Cassano, Pamela Keel, Wade H. Berrettini, and Walter H. Kaye. "Personality in Men with Eating Disorders." *Journal of Psychosomatic Research* 57 (September 2004): 273–78.

World Health Organization World Mental Health Survey Consortium. "Prevalence, Severity, and Unmet Need for Treatment of Mental Disorders in the World Health Organization World Mental Health Surveys." *JAMA: The Journal of the American Medical Association* 291, no. 21 (June 2, 2004): 2581–90.

Zerbe, Kathryn. "Eating Disorders in Middle and Late Life: A Neglected Problem." *Primary Psychiatry* 10 (June 2003): 80–82.

Index

Reading Group Guide

Introduction to the *Gaining* Reading Group Guide

from Aimee Liu

I first decided to write *Gaining* because I was curious. I wanted to see if there was anything to my suspicion that certain personality traits, which seemed to set us up for eating disorders, might still shape our lives in distinct patterns even decades after recovery. I also wanted to find out what scientists know now about eating disorders that they didn't know thirty years ago, when I was first recovering from anorexia. But I wasn't sure how many other people would share my curiosity, and I didn't know that the stories and research I was to study would be so fascinating!

By the time *Gaining* was ready for publication, I knew that I had been profoundly changed by what I'd learned in my research, and I knew that I had never read a book like the one I'd just written. I hoped the stories I'd collected would help others to learn about themselves, as they had helped me; perhaps I was too close to the material, though. I feared the book might get lost among the new nonfiction releases. To be sure, the early review comments from experts in the field of eating disorder treatment and research were tremendously heartening, but what about the families and individuals who had actually wrestled with these illnesses? How would they find their way to this title, and what would they think if and when they read it?

What I didn't fully appreciate was the hunger for new insight into the mysteries of anorexia and bulimia nervosa. Messages began pouring into my in-box as soon as *Gaining* was published. People told me their stories, shared their frustrations and fears, expressed their most urgent hopes. Most of those who wrote were not in the immediate grip of an eating disorder but were caught in the same "half-life" that had held me for nearly thirty years. They had gained control of their eating behavior but still were not free psychologically. They had never connected the dots between their compulsive dieting, bingeing, and purging and their compulsive fitness regimens or vegetarianism, their punishing work habits, problems with trust and sexual intimacy, and the deeply felt (if not necessarily conscious) belief that when the going gets tough, the tough punish themselves. This group shared a common assumption that suffering is an absolute requirement for perfection. And every one of them, to varying degrees, felt driven to be perfect.

I'd like to share a few of these letters with you here, because I think they reflect a range of perspectives and concerns that have been too long neglected. Also, I believe that we gain power by sharing our stories and experiences. Shame and denial too often perpetuate psychological disorders. By sharing truths that we experience as unique we often reach universal insights.

The following are brief excerpts, but they indicate just how much we all have to gain as we become self-aware and "self-centered" in the best of senses.

I am sixteen years old, soon to be seventeen, and since the age of twelve I have struggled tremendously with my weight. I dealt with severe to moderate anorexia until I was fourteen. Then I nearly lost my mother, and could no longer function without physical strength, so I began to eat again. I was successfully "recovered" for several months, but I found the weight gain so hard to bear I slipped into severe depression. I was forced to transfer out of my prestigious prep school to public schooling after my freshman year. It was then that I began my battle with bulimia and have been at it ever since . . . I had no intention of devouring [*Gaining*] as I did because in truth, it's been nearly a year since I've read anything aside from *Vanity Fair* in full (I am unable to focus due to my inconsistent diet and depression). When I read the first few pages my heart leapt to my throat. To find someone . . . who empathized with the true emotional torment of EDs but had learned to live despite it—you gave me hope.

—Connecticut

After pregnancy had, I thought, cured me of eating disorders, my anorexia resurfaced shortly after Hurricane Katrina. I stopped eating when it became clear that we were going to be displaced for a while, and I lost more than ten pounds during the six weeks of our evacuation in Houston. Your book is really helping me to see that many things I thought were completely unrelated to my food issues are connected . . . I've already spoken with one of my aunts about the history on my mother's side of the family and have a call in to another aunt to discuss my father's side of the family. My mother's sister had no idea that I'd experienced eating disorders, and it was very liberating to talk about it with her.

—Louisiana

When you spoke of nail biting and anxiety and hiding behind a computer so you didn't have to speak to your husband, it was if I was looking in the mirror. My major conversations with my husband take place via e-mail. I love the man to death and I know he loves me, but I am afraid to talk to him about things that bother me. My fear of his disapproval is so strong that I can't fight through it. I want to have the perfect household, where everyone is content and happy. I stuff my anger and frustrations and eventually end up punishing myself for them . . . I need to move on with the better half of my life, because I know the alternative to that is death, and I do have too much to live for. I will tell myself this every day for as long as it takes.

—Michigan

My wife has started to read your book . . . She grew up in a good home, with good parents, yet found herself to be the only one of three kids who went down the path of drugs to anorexia to bulimia to defeating all of those actions years later . . . We were married three years ago, and I knew nothing about eating disorders or the psychological issues that promote them . . . Everything was fine while we were dating; then when we got engaged things started to slide and continue to slide up to today. By "slide" I mean that she has gradually pulled farther and farther away from any form of intimacy . . . Being married to someone who can't enter into intimacy is really, really tough and I often think about divorce, not because I don't love her, but because she won't let me be her husband and she won't let herself be my wife . . . I find myself reaching out for her only to be rejected with a blank stare.

—California

I'm fifty-nine years old. I appear successful at a writing vocation, marriage, and emotional health. I have accomplished a lot coming from the family I came from, but anorexia has returned to nip at me. Eating-disordered thinking with all its different behaviors had been a part of my life since my teens. I've never been hospitalized but I was in outpatient groups and spent years in therapy. I thought I was over it, though I recognized how rules and believing in "perfect" still dominated my life. I overcame so much to get where I am. My husband's health began to deteriorate several years ago, which he has faced quite bravely, and I also got breast cancer (which luckily was caught in the early stages). My anxiety kept growing and my restricting grew apace. I felt crazed—what was going on? How could I be so troubled at my age with all the luck and goodness in my life? I found a therapist, highly experienced . . . I've been seeing her privately and in a group too. The group is composed of women forty-five and over and breaks my bewildering isolation . . . Now, at last, I have real evidence that I can feel my feelings, make mistakes, and be at peace with less than sublime—even be "ordinary".

—Washington

Our son, eighteen, has been struggling with AN/BN for almost four years, has been hospitalized multiple times, has done partial hospitalization programs, residential programs for emotionally fragile adolescents, etc. He is supported by great people in school, great ED physician, psychiatrist, therapist, nutritionist, family therapist, you name it. I've realized that all of this "therapy" has not addressed what you described in the introduction as the knowing yourself stage but instead focused on the second and third stages . . . I thought that you expressed so well what it is that has held [my son] hostage all this time and helped me to define a path in my own mind for recovery that makes sense.

—Massachusetts

These letters remind me how important it is to "connect the dots," not only within our own private experience, but also in our experiences with each other. Eating disorders act to isolate us, but in fact, none of us is isolated. We all have partners, parents, children, friends, and colleagues who are deeply concerned and affected by our struggles. Many of them are eager to help, if only given a chance. I hope this book will help to forge those larger connections, as well as help each of us to better understand ourselves.

—Aimee Liu

Questions to Enrich Your Reading of *Gaining: The Truth About Life After Eating Disorders*

1. The author attempts to "connect the dots" to create a complete and understandable picture of eating disorders. What are the "dots" she refers to?

2. Did your own picture of eating disorders change after reading this book? How, and why?

3. In the introduction, Dr. Joel Yager says, "Know thyself in a very profound Greek way. What is your biology? What is your calling? How are you built? Study your temperament. Be respectful of it." This book stresses the importance of self-awareness as a key to mental health. Do you agree with this emphasis? Do you think this advice is specific to those with histories of eating disorders?

4. In chapter 3, the author describes being stunned to realize that perfectionism is the exception rather than the rule among high achievers. Were you surprised by the results of the study that proved this to her? What do you think the true requirements are for high achievement—for example, in school?

5. In chapter 4, former nun Karen Armstrong describes the anorexia that proliferated in her convent as a form of bodily rebellion "against the religious regime we had endured." What forces within a convent might promote eating disorders? Do you consider religion to be a contributing factor or a source of protection against these disorders?

6. In chapter 6, the metaphor of a gun is used to describe how genetics, environment, and emotional experience interact to produce an eating disorder. Do you think this is an apt metaphor? Could it be used to describe other mental or physical conditions, or is it somehow unique to eating disorders?

7. Chapter 6 includes the story of a man who has struggled with anorexia nervosa. A Harvard study released after the initial publication of *Gaining* found that 25 percent of people with anorexia and/or bulimia are male. Does this surprise you? Why or why not?

8. Chapters 7 and 8 discuss the roles of family dynamics and parenting in the development of eating disorders. What do you think are the most important steps parents can take to protect their children?

9. Chapter 10 highlights the critical distinctions between compulsion and passion. What do you think are the most important distinctions? Do you think that you operate more out of compulsion or out of passion?

10. The title word "gaining" has multiple meanings here. Which do you find the most profound for your own life? Why? After finishing the book, what do you feel you have gained?

11. Given what you've learned from this book, do you think it is possible to prevent eating disorders? If you were to become an activist in the fight against eating disorders, what are some of the specific actions you would take?